ESSENTIAL GUT HEALTH FOR WOMEN OVER 50

A STEP-BY-STEP GUIDE TO STABILIZE YOUR DIGESTIVE SYSTEM, CREATE HORMONAL BALANCE WHILE BOOSTING YOUR MOOD

J.L. SERVICE

TABLE OF CONTENTS

INTRODUCTION

UNVEILING THE PATH TO OPTIMAL GUT HEALTH FOR WOMEN OVER 50

"Every day we live and every meal we eat, we influence the great microbial organ inside us – for better or for worse."

— *GIULIA ENDERS*

The gut: a complex and awe-inspiring ecosystem within us that silently orchestrates our overall well-being. Its significance extends beyond digestion, pivotal in our physical health, mental clarity, and emotional balance. For women over 50, maintaining a vibrant and resilient gut becomes increasingly crucial, directly impacting the quality of life during this transformative phase.

I embarked on a remarkable journey that led me to explore the depths of gut health after a series of events shook the very core of my being. Three rounds of antibiotics, once prescribed to heal, inadvertently disrupted the delicate harmony within my gastrointestinal realm. What followed was a profound shift that altered not only my physicality but also my identity and daily experiences.

The repercussions were staggering—constant discomfort plagued my days as bloating, gas, and relentless headaches became unwelcome companions. Even the simplest pleasures, like enjoying a glass of wine, became a source of distress as my body struggled to process alcohol. I was a shadow of my former self, robbed of vitality and joie de vivre. Desperate for relief, I sought refuge in the healing embrace of a gut restoration program offered by a wellness spa.

Within the sanctuary of the spa, I was introduced to a revelation that would reshape my understanding of health—my gut microbiome was imbalanced, lacking the vital diversity required for optimal functioning. The "bad" bacteria had taken over, stifling the growth of their beneficial counterparts and wreaking havoc on my entire system. Armed with newfound knowledge, I dedicated myself to restoring the harmony within, nurturing, and revitalizing my gut ecosystem.

This book is the culmination of my personal odyssey—an empowering resource meticulously crafted to guide women over 50 toward reclaiming their gut health and, subsequently, their lives. It delves into the intricate workings of the gut microbiome, unraveling the profound connection between our inner ecology and overall well-being. Drawing upon the latest scientific research, expert insights, and experiences, I present a comprehensive roadmap towards a thriving gut and unlocking a renewed sense of vitality.

Within these pages, you will discover:

- The vital role of gut health in women over 50 and its impact on overall wellness
- The intricate relationship between the gut and common ailments experienced during this life stage
- Practical strategies to restore and maintain a diverse and resilient gut microbiome
- Nourishing dietary principles tailored to the specific needs of women over 50
- Mind-body practices that harmonize the gut-brain axis and promote emotional equilibrium

- Strategies for managing stress, improving sleep, and enhancing mental clarity
- The transformative power of self-care and its profound influence on gut health

Through this holistic approach to gut health, I hope to empower you, dear reader, to embark on your own journey of healing and rejuvenation. Together, we will navigate the intricate terrain of the gut, shedding light on the path towards vibrant health and embracing the fullness of life that awaits us. Let us embark on this transformative voyage, where the gut becomes not just a vessel of digestion but a source of vitality, joy, and resilience.

PART I

WHY YOUR GUT HEALTH IS SO IMPORTANT

UNLEASHING THE POWER WITHIN: THE VITAL SIGNIFICANCE OF YOUR GUT HEALTH

Gut Health Detectives: Unmasking the Covert Operation of Unhappy Microbes... When Your Stomach Sends Morse Code Messages!"

In recent years, having a healthy digestive system has become increasingly important. Since the gut microbiome, or community of bacteria in the stomach, affects practically every aspect of health, from mood to the ability to fight infection, people are looking for simple ways to boost their gut health. It is consequently uncommon for patients with gastrointestinal problems to experience symptoms unrelated to digestion. So how can you tell whether your digestive system needs some TLC (Tender Loving Care)? In what ways does this manifest physically and mentally? Here are some of the most concerning symptoms of digestive system distress.

Gas, bloating, and other stomach issues

Problems with gut bacteria may lie at the root of food intolerance symptoms like bloating, gas, and stomach pain. Trouble breathing, swelling of the mouth and tongue, and itching are all unpleasant and, in extreme cases, life-threatening symptoms. Although only a tiny percentage of the population has life-threatening food allergies, up to 20% of the population may experience discomfort in the digestive tract due to food intolerances. An intolerant individual may feel well after eating a minimal amount of the offending item, even though higher amounts can trigger severe reactions. You may not have healthy intestinal flora if you have unpleasant sensations like gas and bloating after eating.

Unintentional weight fluctuations

Given that a healthy stomach effectively digests food and consistently expels waste, it's not hard to see how your gut health could affect your weight. If you continue eating as usual, your weight won't be a significant concern. However, there is more to the connection between gut health and weight than meets the eye. One's gastrointestinal bacteria may affect how many calories are absorbed from a diet, as researchers have shown a correlation between metabolic rate and gut microbe makeup. The composition of one's gut flora may influence their propensity to acquire or lose weight. Inconsistent weight gain or loss in response to dietary changes has been linked to poor gut health and a restricted microbiome. However, if your weight suddenly and unexpectedly changes without a corresponding shift in your dietary or physical activity patterns, you should immediately make an appointment with your doctor.

Skin Issues/Your skin is acting up.

Skin inflammation can be brought on by external allergens, internal microbial imbalances, or even just the stress of everyday life. It stands to reason that a thriving microbiome would contribute to glowing skin. An altered immune response from an imbalance in the gut microbiota can cause several skin disorders. A diet heavy in processed foods and salt is associated with fluid retention and skin irritation.

For example, if your diet is high in refined sugar and saturated fat, your gut bacteria may respond by triggering acne outbreaks. In addition, an imbalance of gut flora has been linked to various skin conditions, including acne, rosacea, eczema, psoriasis, and dandruff. The connection between the gut and the skin becomes more apparent when comparing the microbiota of people with and without chronic inflammatory skin conditions.

Disturbances in Emotional and Behavioral Regulation

Our GI tract is closely linked to our moods and emotions. As an illustration, the nerves that stimulate the brain are constantly firing when worry or depression cause the brain to go into overdrive. The same holds for the digestive system. This feedback loop is established when the nerves that stimulate the digestive system also begin to fire. Both the psychological and the gastrointestinal symptoms exacerbate each other. This can continue until the cycle ends, usually by the use of medicine, changes in lifestyle, or a change in nutrition. Numerous studies have demonstrated the importance of gut health to one's emotional well-being. For instance, IBS patients are more likely to have melancholy, anxiety, or sleep problems than the general population, and it's not unusual for depression and generalized anxiety disorder to be linked to gastrointestinal disorders. This is because the gastrointestinal tract and the brain communicate with each other.

Fatigue or insomnia

Are you experiencing a combination of not getting enough sleep and staying up too late? The repercussions of digestive distress can manifest in other ways as well. The digestive system produces most of the serotonin that controls mood and sleep. Our circadian rhythms—which govern our eating, sleeping, and emotional states—are influenced by the activity and functions of the gut. Just as we found a symbiotic association between the stomach and mental health, so do we find a symbiotic relationship between sleep and gut health. Sleeping enough hours each night is essential for intestinal wellness. Regular, undisturbed sleep is vital to sustaining a healthy composition of gut microbes. Lack of sleep and abdominal discomfort may become a self-perpetuating cycle.

Sugar Cravings

The genetic histories of microbes and humans are very similar. This is reasonable since various bacteria have unique dietary needs. For example, a high-sugar diet may be ideal for some bacteria, while a diet higher in carbs, fiber, or even specific lipids may be preferable for others. Once the issue of hunger is resolved, it is expected that the bacteria responsible for it will multiply rapidly. Giving in to the sugar-loving, inflammation-promoting bacteria in your stomach could be a huge mistake.

You're inexplicably exhausted.

If you get the recommended amount of sleep each night but still yawn frequently or struggle with common activities, an imbalance in your digestive system may be to blame. This may be related to the difficulties falling asleep due to emotional issues discussed before. Not receiving enough nutrients into the intestines could lead to malabsorption and fatigue. Dullness, heaviness, and forgetfulness are classic signs of disease, often beginning in the stomach. If you're having difficulties sleeping, don't automatically blame your stomach; instead, consider changing your sleep regimen or visiting a doctor.

Your head hurts.

Headaches can occur when problems in the digestive tract prevent nutrients from being absorbed adequately. The gut-brain axis and neuroinflammation may be involved here. Although migraines are more complicated, research has shown that they can cause stomach discomfort. When both migraines and stomach pain occur simultaneously, or when migraine sufferers experience occasional abdominal discomfort without accompanying headaches, they are said to suffer from abdominal migraines. Hormonal imbalances, which can often bring on headaches and migraines, may also lead to digestive problems.

You're constipated or bloated.

Constipation, bloating, and other symptoms of poor gut health may be rooted in microbial imbalances and digestive dysfunction. Distinguishing between a short-term stomachache caused by something you ate and a more serious digestive condition is not always manageable. For example, you may have overeaten the day before if you haven't had to go to the bathroom for more than two days but are still experiencing abdominal distention. Perhaps you filled food or didn't drink enough water. Both gas and constipation typically disappear after a week.

You have bad breath.

Poor oral hygiene is a surprising indicator of gastrointestinal distress. However, this is why it occurs: Toxins can build up in the body if waste isn't eliminated regularly, as in the case of chronic or recurrent constipation. One of the most obvious signs of digestive system distress this can cause is bad breath. Therefore, you should reconsider your diet if your breath still smells terrible despite diligent brushing and flossing.

You're irregular (for you).

Bowel movements are deemed "regular" when they occur at a rate of at least once per three days. A more serious warning that your gut health needs attention is if the fluctuation in frequency causes symptoms or significantly disrupts your typical rhythm. A person's bowel habits should be closely monitored if they experience significant changes.

You have new food sensitivities.

Intestinal problems are another common cause of food allergies. A "leaky gut," in which the cells lining your intestine are permeable, is a common manifestation of this phenomenon. Harvard Health Publishing states that a semi-permeable gut lining is necessary to absorb water and nutrients from food into the bloodstream. However, increased permeability can occur when intercellular spaces become abnormally large or lax. As a result, inflammation can develop from entering large food particles and microorganisms into the circulation. This may play a role in developing food sensitivities, including gastrointestinal (GI) symptoms like diarrhea, bloating, gas, constipation, nausea, and extra-GI symptoms, including headaches, brain fog, and skin rashes.

In the tapestry of our lives, the gut stands as a silent champion, tirelessly working behind the scenes to support us in every endeavor. From physical vitality to mental clarity, emotional balance to immune resilience, our gut health influences the very fabric of our existence. And for women over 50, the significance of nurturing and managing our gut health becomes even more pronounced. It is a key to unlocking the fullness of life during this transformative phase. By cultivating an awareness of our gut's profound impact on every aspect of our being, we gain the power to actively manage and nurture this essential ecosystem. Let us embrace this knowledge with open arms, for within it lies the potential to embark on a journey of profound well-being, where our gut health becomes a guiding force toward a life of vibrancy, purpose, and vitality.

PART II

HOW YOUR DIGESTIVE SYSTEM WORKS

1

YOUR SECOND BRAIN: UNLEASHING THE HIDDEN POWER OF YOUR GUT

Gut Intelligence: When Your Stomach Becomes a Mastermind, and Your Brain Goes on Lunch Break!

The digestive system's complex network of neurons, neurotransmitters, and other substances has earned it the nickname "second brain" due to its ability to function independently and communicate with the brain. The enteric nervous system (ENS) is a network of nerve cells that lines the gastrointestinal tract from the esophagus to the rectum. The ENS may take over and take care of things if the central nervous system (CNS) isn't involved. Among the various digestive processes demonstrated to be affected by this hormone are food movement, digestive enzyme and hormone synthesis, and gastrointestinal blood flow. The ENS is not necessary for digestion and influences our moods, thoughts, and the quality of our decision-making.

The ENS produces and responds to neurotransmitters like serotonin, dopamine, and GABA, which regulate mood and behavior. Science has proven that the vagus nerve, which runs from the base of the brain to the lower belly, connects the ENS to the CNS. The gut-brain axis is a two-way communication route linked to one's emotional health, stress levels, and immune response. The digestive system is often called the "second brain" because of the complex network of neurons, neurotransmitters, and hormones that enable it to perform its own functions and engage in two-way communication with the brain. Through the gut-brain axis, the enteric nervous system (ENS) controls digestion, influences our emotions, and communicates with the central nervous system (CNS).

THE DIGESTIVE SYSTEM

The GI tract, often known as the digestive system, comprises the pancreas, liver, and gallbladder. The digestive system (GI) is a tube-like collection of hollow organs that travels from the mouth to the genitalia via several twists and turns. Tube-shaped organs such as the mouth, stomach, small intestine, large intestine, esophagus, and anus make up the digestive system. Three solid organs—the gallbladder, liver, and pancreas —make up the digestive system. The small intestine can be roughly divided into three distinct parts. The first part, the duodenum, is the first digestive tract. The jejunum and the ileum are at either end of the digestive tract. All of these parts—the appendix, cecum, colon, and rectum—makeup what we call the large intestine. The appendix is a small pouch the size of a finger that sits near the cecum. The cecum is the initial part of the large intestine. Next up is the colon. The rectum is the remaining portion of the big intestine.

The Digestive System

Photo credit: NIH.gov

The digestion of food and drink is crucial to the proper functioning and maintenance of your body. Protein, fat, carbohydrate, vitamin, mineral, and water are all examples of nutrients. Nutrients must break down into ever-tinier particles for the body to absorb and use them for energy, development, and cell repair.

- Proteins are constructed from amino acids.
- Free fatty acids and glycerol are produced when fats are metabolized.
- Starches are broken down into sugars.

What happens to food as it travels through the digestive system?

We should be discussing "your second brain."

The digestive tract can move food forward thanks toperistalsis. There are several large, hollow organs in your digestive system, each lined with muscle so that it can move. This action helps move food and drink through your digestive system and mixes the contents of your organs. When one muscle contracts and squeezes food forward, another muscle relaxes, causing the food to be propelled forward.

Mouth. After a meal, digestion begins as food travels through the digestive tract. Food is guided down the esophagus with the help of the tongue. The epiglottis is a little flap of tissue that closes over the windpipe to block food from entering the esophagus and causing choking.

Esophagus. Swallowing becomes a habit that is hard to break. The process of peristalsis begins when the brain sends a signal to the muscles of the esophagus.

Lower esophageal sphincter. A ring-shaped muscle at the very end of the esophagus, called the lower esophageal sphincter, simply relaxes to allow food to pass into the stomach. This sphincter is normally closed to prevent the reflux of stomach acid into the esophagus.

Stomach. The stomach's muscular lining incorporates the contents of the stomach into digestive juices. Chyme, the stomach's contents, makes its way into the small intestine very slowly.

Small intestine. The small intestine's muscles push food through the digestive system, where it mixes with digestive juices produced by the pancreas, liver, and gut. The intestinal mucosa, which is very small, absorbs fluids and nutrients from the digested food and sends them into the bloodstream. As digestion continues, waste products are moved into the large intestine via peristalsis.

Large intestine. The digestive process produces waste products such as fluid, undigested food, and dead cells from the gastrointestinal system lining. The large intestine uses water from the waste to create stools. With the help of peristalsis, the stool is forced into the rectum.

Rectum. The rectum is part of your large intestine that collects waste until it is time for a bowel movement, pushing the waste out of your anus.

How do my digestive organs break down food into digestible chunks?

As food enters your digestive system, your organs attempt to pulverize it.

- Biting, squeezing, and stirring are all examples of motion.
- Digestive juices (including enzymes, bile, and water)

Mouth. When you chew, your body releases digestive enzymes, and the process begins. Your salivary glands produce saliva, a digestive juice that helps break down food and facilitates swallowing and digestion. Saliva contains an enzyme that swiftly breaks down the starch in your food.

Esophagus. When you swallow, a coordinated contraction of your esophagus and stomach takes place; this is called peristalsis.

Stomach. Glands in the stomach lining secrete acid and digestive enzymes. Stomach muscles work to combine meals and digestive juices.

Pancreas. The digestive juice your pancreas secretes contains enzymes that aid in breaking carbs, fats, and proteins. Pancreatic digestive juices enter the small intestine through ducts to kick off the digestion process.

Liver. The liver produces bile, a digestive fluid that is crucial for the digestion of fats and even some vitamins. Bile is delivered from the liver to the small intestine and the gallbladder via the bile ducts.

Gallbladder. The gallbladder acts as a reservoir for bile between meals. The gallbladder receives and stores bile, which is then released into the small intestine at the appropriate time.

Small intestine. The small intestine secretes digestive juice, which collaborates with bile and pancreatic juice to aid in the digestion of lipids, proteins, and carbohydrates. The bacteria in your small intestine make digestive enzymes that help you digest food. The small intestine pulls water from the bloodstream and pumps it into the digestive system. Water and nutrients are absorbed at the same time in the small intestine.

Large intestine. The area around the large intestine is particularly well-suited for water absorption from the digestive tract into the bloodstream. Bacteria in the large intestine produce vitamin K, a beneficial digestive enzyme. Vitamin K is also produced in the early stages of digestion. The stool consists of undigested food remnants and other waste items.

After digestion, where does all that food go?

The small intestine is responsible for breaking down most of the food you ingest, and the nutrients are then distributed throughout the body via the blood. Nutrients are absorbed when certain cells transport them over the intestinal mucosa and into the bloodstream. Glucose, amino acids, glycerol, and other vitamins and minerals are all transported to the liver via the blood. The liver is responsible for processing, storing, and distributing nutrition. The lymph system is a network of veins that transports white blood cells and lymph fluid throughout the body to aid in immune defense, nutrient uptake, and fatty acid use. Carbohydrates, amino acids, fatty acids, and glycerol are all used by the body for energy, growth, and cell repair.

THE ROLE OF PROPER DIGESTION IN MAINTAINING GENERAL HEALTH

Contrary to popular perception, gut microbiota has been found to have significant impacts on human health. The microbiome, or collection of gut bacteria, is crucial to your health and evolves with time. Your gut microorganisms are more beneficial to your health if they come from a wide variety of sources.

Helpful Germs

You host a wide variety of microorganisms. They far outnumber your own cells. The ones found in the digestive tract are crucial for digesting food and may have positive effects on your mind and body.

Gut Microbiome

The community of bacteria, yeasts, and viruses that makes it home in our digestive tracts helps break down food so your body can absorb the nutrients it needs.

Fighting the Good Fight

It's not simply digestion that benefits from the "good" bacteria that populate the gut microbiome. They help keep "bad" germs under control. The high reproduction rate of the unfit strain causes its eventual eradication.

The body feels at ease when there is a healthy mix of microorganisms in the digestive tract.

Unhealthy Balance

The presence of a certain type of pathogenic bacteria in the gut microbiome has been linked to an increased risk of developing the following illnesses:

- Crohn's disease
- Irritable bowel syndrome (IBS)
- Ulcerative colitis

Gut Bacteria and Your Heart

Bacteria in the gut may have an impact on the relationship between cholesterol and cardiovascular disease. Bacteria in meals like red meat and eggs create the chemical trimethylamine-N-oxide (TMAO). TMAO may facilitate the production of arterial cholesterol. DMB is a molecule that has been the focus of intensive scientific study. It is present in both olive and grapeseed oils. Researchers think it has the potential to inhibit TMAO formation by your bacteria. Eating more fruit, legumes, and vegetables, taking more vitamins, D and B, eating more pistachios and Brussels sprouts, and taking probiotics can help lower TAMO levels.

Gut Bacteria and Your Kidneys

TMAO overdose can potentially cause chronic renal dysfunction. Patients with this condition have problems flushing out TMAO. TMAO surplus raises the danger of cardiovascular disease. Researchers found that high levels of TMAO were associated with chronic renal disease.

Gut Bacteria and Your Brain

Messages sent from the brain travel throughout the entire body. Some studies have suggested that your belly might convey information to you. Scientists have discovered that an individual's gut microbiome can affect their mental state and how their brain processes sensory information. Researchers believe that changes to this balance play a role in the emergence of autism spectrum disorder, anxiety, despair, and chronic pain.

THE VAGUS NERVE AND THE NERVOUS SYSTEM

Neurons are specialized brain and nervous system cells responsible for directing behavior. The vagus nerve is a major nerve that communicates between the digestive system and the brain.

Neurotransmitters

Neurotransmitters, like serotonin, are brain molecules that regulate our emotional states. The cells and bacteria in the digestive tract create neurotransmitters like gamma-aminobutyric acid (GABA).

Gut microbes produce additional brain-affecting chemicals.

Gut microorganisms produce short-chain fatty acids (SCFA) like butyrate, propionate, and acetate. These SCFAs have multiple effects on brain activity, including suppressing hunger and helping to structure the blood-brain barrier. Other compounds that affect the brain are produced through the metabolism of bile acids and amino acids.

Gut Bacteria and Obesity

If the balance of your gut flora is off, your brain may send mixed messages about whether or not you are hungry or full. Since the pituitary gland secretes satiety hormones, it has been theorized that it plays a role. The microorganisms in the stomach can have their makeup changed by this gland as well. Some research into obesity therapies aims to draw this link.

YOU CAN CHANGE YOUR GUT BACTERIA

Your gut microbiota is mainly determined by your genetic composition and the environment you were exposed to before and after birth. The foods you eat can also have an effect.

Probiotics

Good microorganisms that reside in the gut are called probiotics. Your body already contains "good" bacteria comparable to certain foods. They can boost the beneficial bacteria in your digestive system, making you feel more at peace with yourself. They're not all the same, though. There is a wide variety, each with its unique mode of action and potential side effects.

How Can Probiotics Help?

They can strengthen your immune system so it can better fight off disease. They may help soothe irritable bowel syndrome and other gastrointestinal issues. Some probiotics may help with both lactose intolerance and allergic responses. However, this effectiveness is highly dependent on the gut microbiota composition.

Sources of Probiotics

Probiotics can be found in various dairy products, including yogurt and aged cheeses. Live bacteria, like bifidobacteria and lactobacilli, should be listed as an ingredient if the product claims to have probiotic health benefits. They can also be found in pickled vegetables like onions and gherkins and fermented vegetables like kimchi and sauerkraut.

Prebiotics

Prebiotics are compounds in food that foster the growth of beneficial bacteria. Prebiotics feed the good bacteria (microorganisms They are typically found in plant-based foods, such as fruits and vegetables.

- Asparagus
- Bananas
- Onions
- Soybeans
- Leeks
- Garlic
- Artichokes

They are also found in dishes made with whole wheat.

Synbiotics

Synbiotics are a mixture of probiotics and prebiotics that beneficially affects us by improving the survival of the beneficial bacteria. Prebiotics help probiotics work better by feeding the good bacteria already present in the gut. When combined, they have a mutually beneficial effect. The intent is to prolong the life of probiotics. Asparagus and tempeh in a stir-fry, or bananas and yogurt, are two examples of delicious synbiotic food combinations. Synbiotics are products in which the prebiotic compounds selectively from the growth of the probiotics.

GUT HEALTH AND MENOPAUSE

The significance of the gut microbiota in the changes in body composition and metabolic risk factors found in postmenopausal women is still poorly understood, even though the gut microbiota plays a vital regulatory role in metabolism and modulates estrogen metabolism.

These findings emphasize the need for more investigation into the role of the gut microbiota in metabolic and structural changes associated with menopause, which could lead to new treatments. The increased metabolic risk that postmenopausal women experience may be due to changes in the microbiota, which are vital to systemic and estrogenic metabolism. The microbiome may provide a novel approach to reducing metabolic risk during menopause.

How the gut/brain axis can change your mood and even personality

The bacteria in your gut produce many of the neurotransmitters that are essential for your brain, mood, and mental health. Most of your body's supply of serotonin also called the "happy" chemical or hormone, is made in your digestive system. Serotonin is mainly produced in the intestines (about 90%). The bacteria in your gut play a role in this by sending signals to stimulate serotonin production. Dopamine, gamma-aminobutyric acid, and norepinephrine are neurotransmitters produced in the stomach that contribute to mood and mental wellness.

HORMONES AND GUT HEALTH

Hormonal fluctuations, especially the decline in estrogen levels, can affect the composition and functioning of the gut microbiota. Estrogen receptors are present throughout the gut, and these hormones play a role in maintaining the integrity of the intestinal lining, regulating gut motility, and modulating immune responses.

Here are a few ways in which hormones and gut health interact in women over 50:

- Digestive issues: Fluctuating hormone levels can impact digestive processes, leading to bloating, gas, constipation, or diarrhea. Estrogen helps regulate bowel movements, and a decline in its levels may contribute to irregularities in gut motility.
- Gut microbiota changes: Estrogen influences the composition of gut bacteria, promoting a healthy balance of beneficial microbes. As estrogen levels decline, there may be changes in the gut microbiome, potentially affecting digestion, nutrient absorption, and immune function.
- Increased risk of gut disorders: Postmenopausal women may be more susceptible to certain gastrointestinal conditions, including irritable bowel syndrome (IBS) and inflammatory bowel disease (IBD). These conditions are thought to be influenced by hormonal changes and gut microbiota alterations.
- Bone health connection: While not directly related to gut health, it's worth mentioning that estrogen plays a crucial role in maintaining bone density. Hormonal changes during menopause can increase the risk of osteoporosis, which may also indirectly affect gut health.

Maintaining gut health in women over 50:

- Balanced diet: A nutrient-rich, high-fiber diet supports a healthy gut. Include a variety of fruits, vegetables, whole grains, and fermented foods like yogurt or sauerkraut to promote beneficial gut bacteria.
- Probiotics and prebiotics: Consider incorporating probiotic-rich foods or supplements into your routine to support the growth of beneficial gut microbes. Prebiotics nourish these microbes and are found in foods like onions, garlic, and bananas.
- Regular exercise: Physical activity can help support digestion and overall well-being. Exercise has been linked to a diverse gut microbiota and improved gut function.
- Stress management: Chronic stress can negatively impact gut health. Explore stress-reducing techniques such as meditation, deep breathing exercises, or engaging in hobbies you enjoy.
- Hormone replacement therapy (HRT): Discuss with your healthcare provider whether hormone replacement therapy is appropriate for you. HRT may help manage menopause

symptoms and alleviate gut-related issues by stabilizing hormone levels.

Hormones: A Natural Method for Balancing Them

For both menstrual and postmenopausal women, focusing on the gut and returning to the fundamentals of health can give great relief. Diet, rest, physical activity, stress reduction, and probiotics are the new weapons in the fight against female hormonal imbalance. Let's check out each of these all-natural approaches to hormone regulation.

Balance Hormones with Diet

By promoting digestive health, guaranteeing adequate levels of micronutrients, and managing blood sugar, a whole-food, anti-inflammatory diet that includes healthy fat can aid in hormone synthesis. Naturally, the diet needs to be tailored to the individual, and any potentially allergenic items should be avoided. Refined carbohydrates, sugar, processed foods, and inflammatory lipids are all drastically reduced on an anti-inflammatory diet.

- Meat
- Dairy products
- Whole grains
- Fruits

- Vegetables
- Fish
- Nuts
- Seeds

Dietary Fat

Dietary fats are an essential component of a healthy diet and play a crucial role in the overall well-being of women over 50. While choosing the right types and quantities of fats is important, incorporating healthy fats into your diet can offer several benefits. Here are some key advantages of dietary fats for women over 50:

In hormone regulation: Fats are involved in producing and balancing hormones. Women going through menopause may experience hormonal fluctuations, and consuming adequate healthy fats can help support hormonal balance during this stage of life.

Nutrient absorption: Certain vitamins and minerals, such as vitamins A, D, E, and K, are fat-soluble, requiring fats for absorption. By including healthy fats in your meals, you enhance the absorption of these vital nutrients, promoting overall health.

Heart health: Contrary to earlier misconceptions, not all fats are bad for cardiovascular health. Healthy fats, such as monounsaturated fats and omega-3 fatty acids, can improve heart health by reducing inflammation, lowering LDL (bad) cholesterol levels, and increasing HDL (good) cholesterol levels. This can reduce the risk of heart disease, which becomes increasingly important as women age.

Brain function and cognitive health: The brain mainly comprises fat, and dietary fats are crucial in maintaining optimal brain function. Omega-3 fatty acids, in particular, have been associated with improved cognitive function and a reduced risk of cognitive decline and age-related conditions such as Alzheimer's disease.

Joint health: Healthy fats possess anti-inflammatory properties, which can help alleviate joint pain and stiffness commonly associated with conditions like arthritis. Omega-3 fatty acids, found in fatty fish, walnuts, and flaxseeds, have been shown to have anti-inflammatory effects and may help reduce joint inflammation.

Satiety and weight management: Including healthy fats in your meals can contribute to feelings of fullness and satisfaction after eating. This can help regulate appetite and potentially prevent overeating, supporting weight management goals.

Skin and hair health: Essential fatty acids, such as omega-3 and omega-6, are necessary for maintaining healthy skin and promoting a vibrant complexion.

These fats contribute to skin elasticity, hydration, and protection against oxidative damage. Additionally, they can help nourish the scalp and promote healthy hair growth.

When incorporating dietary fats into your diet, focus on including the following healthy sources:

- Avocados
- Nuts and seeds (e.g., almonds, walnuts, chia seeds, flaxseeds)
- Fatty fish (e.g., salmon, mackerel, sardines)
- Olive oil and other plant-based oils (e.g., coconut oil, flaxseed oil)
- Nut butters (e.g., almond butter, peanut butter)
- Full-fat dairy products (e.g., Greek yogurt, cheese)
- Legumes (e.g., lentils, chickpeas)

As with any nutrient, moderation is key. While healthy fats offer numerous benefits, it's essential to consume them in appropriate portions to maintain a balanced diet and calorie intake. Consulting with a registered dietitian or healthcare professional can provide personalized guidance and help you create a dietary plan that meets your needs.

Menopause and Iron

Menopause and iron levels: Menopause leads to a decrease in estrogen levels, which can affect iron metabolism. After menopause, women no longer have monthly menstrual bleeding, which reduces iron loss. However, iron absorption may be compromised due to age-related changes in the gastrointestinal tract. Therefore, assessing iron status is important to determine whether supplementation is necessary.

Iron deficiency and anemia: Iron deficiency is a common condition, particularly in women. If left untreated, it can progress to iron-deficiency anemia, characterized by low hemoglobin levels and reduced oxygen-carrying capacity. Symptoms of iron-deficiency anemia include fatigue, weakness, shortness of breath, and pale skin. If blood tests indicate iron deficiency or anemia, iron supplementation may be recommended.

- Quinoa
- Leafy greens
- Fish and seafood
- Legumes (lentils and chickpeas)
- Molasses
- Dark chocolate

Zinc can be found naturally in foods, including meat, fish, and seafood. In most circumstances, enough levels of micronutrients can be obtained from eating a balanced diet. When a person consumes a nutritious diet but still has trouble absorbing nutrients, it may be a sign of poor gut health. The priority should be on restoring gut health to increase absorption rather than taking supplements.

Balance Hormones with Sleep

Getting enough sleep is central for everyone's health, but it's especially central for those dealing with the symptoms of hormone imbalance. Menopausal symptoms, including hot flashes, night sweats, restless limb syndrome, and breathing problems, can have a significant effect on a person's ability to sleep and quality of life. Getting into the habit of going to bed and waking up at the same time each day, and sleeping in a cool, dark room without any lights on, is the first step toward improving your quality of life. Also, try to avoid too much screen time right before you turn it in.

Regulate Hormones with Exercise

Another cornerstone of health is physical activity. Spending time in nature, especially in the company of a friend, can help you create a more favorable internal climate for the growth of beneficial bacteria in your gut microbiota. You should work out regularly, but not excessively. Walk for 30 minutes a couple times a week (preferably in a wooded area) if you're just starting off with exercise or getting back into shape after a long period of inactivity. Whether it's weightlifting, swimming, or biking, your workouts can benefit from increasing in intensity and duration as you gain strength. In terms of hormonal manifestations:

- Menopause, constipation, breast tenderness, anxiety, and irritability can all benefit from regular exercise.
- 14 out of 17 menopause symptoms were reduced when swimming compared to women who didn't swim.
- Personalized exercise enhances hormones, maintains healthy blood sugar levels, reduces fatigue by strengthening mitochondria, and promotes restful sleep.

Managing stress and hormone balance

Whether it's the physical kind (from things like over-training and gut dysbiosis to physical trauma) or the emotional kind (from things like anxiety and depression), stress is never fun. If you are unhappy at work or in a challenging relationship, your body may start producing stress hormones like cortisol and adrenaline instead of sex hormones like estrogen, progesterone, and testosterone.

Stress reduction is a vital lifestyle strategy for reestablishing normal hormone levels. Some of the most efficient methods of stress management are also the simplest and least expensive: deep breathing, mindful movement, and meditation.

GUT HEALTH AND MENTAL HEALTH ARE LINKED

Depressive symptoms are linked to "bad" intestinal bacteria, and inflammation.

Gut microbiome variety is important for health because it contributes to microbiome stability. However, when it is not functioning properly (a condition known as dysbiosis), harmful microorganisms can thrive and trigger inflammation. Inflammation occurs after your immune system reacts to the presence of aggressive bacteria. It's interesting to note that depression can trigger inflammation, and inflammation can lead to depression. Anti-inflammatory effects of a varied microbiota, therefore, reducing inflammation can aid in lifting both mood and anxiety. Changing one's diet is one way to increase beneficial gut bacteria, reduce inflammation, and improve overall health.

Butyrate, a short-chain fatty acid, is produced by certain beneficial gut bacteria during the fermentation of dietary fiber. It plays a crucial role in supporting gut health and has been linked to the modulation of psychological well-being. Here's how the butyrate effect on gut microbes and psychological well-being is interconnected:

Gut microbial balance: Butyrate acts as a fuel source for the cells lining the colon and helps maintain their health and integrity. It also supports a healthy balance of gut microbiota by inhibiting the growth of harmful bacteria and promoting the growth of beneficial bacteria. A diverse and balanced gut microbiome is associated with improved gut health and overall well-being.

Gut barrier function: Butyrate plays a role in enhancing the integrity of the gut barrier, which prevents the passage of harmful substances from the intestines into the bloodstream. A healthy gut barrier is important for preventing inflammation and maintaining immune function. Disruption of the gut barrier has been linked to various gastrointestinal disorders and has also been implicated in the development of mental health conditions.

Communication between the gut and brain: The gut and brain are connected through the gut-brain axis, a bidirectional communication system. Butyrate and other metabolites produced by gut bacteria can influence this communication. Butyrate has been shown to have anti-inflammatory effects and can modulate the release of neurotransmitters and neuropeptides that impact mood and cognitive function.

Psychological well-being: Research suggests that an imbalance in gut microbiota, known as dysbiosis, may contribute to the development of mental health conditions such as depression and anxiety. Butyrate's effects on gut health and the gut-brain axis are believed to play a role in influencing psychological well-being. By supporting a healthy gut environment, butyrate may help mitigate inflammation, improve neurotransmitter function, and positively impact mood and mental health.

Potential therapeutic implications: The beneficial effects of butyrate on gut health and psychological well-being have led to investigations into its therapeutic potential. Studies have explored the use of butyrate supplementation or interventions that promote the growth of butyrate-producing bacteria as a means of improving mental health outcomes. However, further research is needed to establish the optimal strategies and dosages for such interventions.

It's important to note that while butyrate appears to have positive effects on gut health and psychological well-being, it is just one piece of the complex puzzle. Maintaining overall good nutrition, a balanced diet rich in fiber, regular physical activity, stress management, and a healthy lifestyle are all important factors in supporting gut health and psychological well-being.

Probiotics and Depression

The brain is just one of the numerous organs that benefit from probiotic microorganisms. They can be found in fermented foods like kefir and yogurt, as well as in supplements. In addition to helping your body in general, probiotics, including Bifidobacterium, Lactobacillus, and Lactococcus species, can also improve your mental state. Some studies have found that particular strains of Lactobacillus help people deal better with stress and reduce anxiety. In some research, taking probiotics has been linked to a reduction in depressive symptoms. Probiotics benefit health by maintaining a healthy microbiome and warding off dysbiosis. By doing so, you increase the chances of butyrate production and the growth of healthy bacteria.

CONSUME PREBIOTICS TO SUPPORT YOUR GUT MICROBES

Studies have also connected prebiotic consumption to improvements in anxiety and related behaviors. Therefore, it is impossible to overestimate the significance of eating well for one's mental health.

Gut microorganisms control the release of endorphins.

Gut microorganisms make short-chain fatty acids (SCFAs) from food, and these SCFAs then interact with the cells that produce serotonin, a neurotransmitter that regulates mood. Some probiotic gut bacteria can create GABA, a neurotransmitter that regulates and enhances mood. By providing them with the fuel they need, the bacteria in your gut will be better able to generate molecules that promote mood-lifting neuro-transmitters like serotonin and GABA, protecting your mental health.

The makeup of your microbiome and your state of mind

There is undeniably a connection between the microbes in your gut and mental health issues like depression. What's going on within a person's body can be gleaned from their gut microbiome's makeup. Keep in mind that everyone has a somewhat different gut flora, but this diversity actually helps maintain a healthy body and mind. The good news is that at-home testing for microbiome health has become increasingly accessible. Find out how well your microbiome produces butyrate, how diverse it is, and what you should eat to maintain a thriving microbiome.

Do at-home testing for microbiome health.

Stool samples are used for microbiome analysis in both clinical and at-home settings. These tests are fecal and require fresh stool samples, as opposed to other types that you may be able to undertake at home using blood or saliva samples. You will need a tool kit like the one below:

- https://www.cerascreen.co.uk/products/gut-microbiome-test

THE ROLE OF GUT BACTERIA IN WEIGHT MANAGEMENT

How Gut Bacteria Can Help You Lose Weight

The microbiome in our intestines comprises billions of beneficial microbes that form an ecosystem vital to our bodily functions, and its composition is correlated with our weight. Dysbiosis occurs in the gut when either the variety of good bacteria or the number of harmful bacteria (or both) decreases. Consequences for health are a real possibility, and understanding the factors that make some people put on weight more quickly than others. Both diet and physical activity can affect the kind of bacteria that live in a person's intestines.

Is there really such a thing as weight-loss microbes?

Some bacteria, like Christensenella Minute and Akkermansia muciniphila, have been related to preventing weight gain and are commonly present in slender people, making them useful for weight loss. Prebiotic foods provide them with the fuel they need to make acetate, a short-chain fatty acid that aids in controlling body fat stores and hunger. Increasing one's consumption of these bacteria may fortify the intestinal lining and protect against weight gain.

Foods to boost Akkermansia

- Flaxseeds
- Cranberries
- Fish oil
- Bamboo shoots
- Concord grapes
- Black tea
- Rhubarb extract

Christensenella is a novel gut bacterium linked to maintaining a healthy weight, and it is commonly present in the microbiomes of slim individuals. This bacterium's association with genetic kinship makes it more common in the digestive systems of people who have a common genetic origin.

Improving your weight loss by altering your gut microbiota

The American Gut Project found that people whose diets included the largest variety of plant items (those with at least 30 distinct colors each week) had the most diverse microbiome.

Plant foods that span the color spectrum are rich in protective phytonutrients like polyphenols, which can neutralize free radicals and reduce inflammation. In addition, they have several beneficial fibers for the digestive system. Both of these things feed the good bacteria that make up the microbiota.

Diet plays a role in both weight gain and gut health.

Overweight people's gut microbiota exhibit dysbiotic patterns, which are linked to inflammation and elevated blood sugar levels, compared to those of healthy people. Following a natural plant-based diet has been demonstrated to minimize calorie intake, speed up weight loss, and decrease metabolic indicators. Patients with type II diabetes who followed a vegan diet had better blood sugar control than those who followed a standard diabetic diet. Better blood sugar regulation has been linked to the presence of helpful bacteria that thrive on plant foods.

Antibiotics, harmful gut flora, and weight gain

Antibiotics promote weight gain because they alter the composition of gut microbes by inhibiting or killing bacteria. Antibiotics are thought to contribute to the rising prevalence of childhood obesity. Early drug use has also been shown to alter the composition of the gut microbiota, which in turn causes metabolic alterations with age.

Many different diseases and disorders, from obesity to mental illness, have been linked to a lack of probiotics in the body. The gut microbiome can be replenished with them, making them useful following a round of antibiotics. The reasoning goes like this: since antibiotics kill out good gut bacteria along with the bad bacteria that could be causing your infection, a probiotic can help put things back in order in your digestive tract.

Maintaining a healthy gut flora and dropping pounds

Walking, running, swimming, cycling, and dancing are all examples of aerobic exercises that increase the number of beneficial bacteria in the intestine and, in turn, lower the risk of dysbiosis by suppressing inflammation and maintaining a healthy gut environment.

The gut microbiome: what happens when you work out?

Physical activity increases muscle energy expenditure and helps maintain healthy levels of metabolic indicators, including blood glucose and lipids. This aids in weight management as well. That's why staying active regularly aids in weight loss and maintenance.

Get healthy gut bacteria by eating the rainbow.

Even though eating a diet rich in fruits, vegetables, and whole grains is critical to good health most people eat less than the suggested 400 gm of fruit and vegetables daily. The lack of these natural plant molecules, known as phytonutrients, is harmful to our health and the helpful gut microorganisms. You may add these foods to your diet with just a little of work.

Eat more rainbow colors to help your body, weight, and gut microbiota, which has been related to weight gain over time.

The truth about gut bacteria and weight loss

There is a strong correlation between gut bacteria and weight gain or loss due to their effects on digestion, fat storage, and appetite. Research reveals no simple solution to altering gut bacteria and slimming them down.

Increasing your intake of plant-based meals, prebiotic fibers, and regular physical activity has been shown to increase the diversity of the gut microbiota and decrease the likelihood of weight gain and obesity. You'll be able to keep the pounds off because inflammation and rising metabolic indicators won't be able to penetrate your gut barrier.

Let's have a peek at what the next chapter covers:

- The Connection Between Mental Health and the Gut
- How does poor gut health affect mental health?
- What is the gut-brain axis?
- How can gut malnutrition affect the brain?
- The gut-brain axis and mental health

2

THE GUT-BRAIN AXIS: THE ASTONISHING CONNECTION BETWEEN YOUR MIND AND GUT

Gut Feelings and Brain Waves: When Your Stomach Drops Knowledge Bombs on Your Nervous System!

What impact does one's Gut have on the brain? Researchers have shown that reducing the number of bacteria in the Gut can have beneficial effects on people's mental health. The microbiome, the complex community of bacteria in your gastrointestinal (GI) tract, is crucial to your overall health and plays a role in everything from skin inflammation to weight gain. Scientists now believe that this capacity to promote wellness extends to the functioning of your brain and nervous system.

What's the Connection?

The thousands of "good" and "bad" bacteria that make up the microbiome often coexist in a healthy equilibrium, with the former helping to keep the latter in check. An imbalance in the microbiome has been linked to inflammation, intestinal permeability, and a lack of bacterial variety, all of which can lead to an overpopulation of harmful bacteria. Researchers sometimes face the age-old "chicken or egg" conundrum when determining the causal order of events between gut microbes and bad health.

How does poor gut health affect mental health?

The body produces its endorphins in the gut, and various neural pathways connect the gut and the brain. They communicate with one another through a series of messages. For example, gas and bloating can make it difficult to rest comfortably at night. However, if your GI system is content, it will signal your brain that all is well. There is a correlation between poor gut health and mental health and vitamin shortages because of the vagus nerve, which connects the brain with the digestive system. In addition to facilitating food transit and stimulating digestive enzyme production, the vagus nerve relays satiety signals to the brain. If you're getting enough nutrients, such as those that help you sleep and think clearly, you don't need to put up with stress and mental suffering. Depression, anxiety, and other mood problems are more likely in people with poor gut health.

Many people are familiar with the connection between the gut and the brain, whether it shows as "butterflies" at the sight of a loved one or nervousness in the stomach before giving a big presentation. The gut-brain axis describes a true phenomenon in which the central nervous system (CNS) and the enteric nervous system (ENS) communicate.

What is the gut-brain axis?

The connection between the gut and the brain is called the "gut-brain axis" because of the two-way communication between the two. The gut becomes linked to the brain's emotional and logical regions. Similar to how a disturbed brain can send signals to a problematic gut, a troubled gut can send signals to a troubled brain. The complex network of numerous routes that facilitates this gut-brain communication is fascinating. Some of them are listed below.

Chemicals produced by gut microbes

One important part of this network is the digestive system, which houses trillions of microbes. One's diet has a significant impact on these microbes. For instance, intestinal bacteria digest dietary fiber to create short-chain fatty acid metabolites. A few examples of these are butyrate, propionate, and acetate. Short-chain fatty acids can change the way the brain is built and how it works since they are able to cross the blood-brain barrier.

Inflammation

The gut-brain axis is a signaling pathway between microbes and the brain, and the immune system plays a crucial role in this pathway. The permeability of the gut-blood barrier is linked to dysbiosis, an imbalance in gut microorganisms. Inflammation may result if "bad" germs are able to infiltrate the bloodstream in this way. Dysbiosis also disrupts the blood-brain barrier, which may cause brain inflammation. Neuroinflammatory ailments, such as Parkinson's disease, Alzheimer's disease, multiple sclerosis, and anxiety and depression-like disorders, have been related to inflammatory pathways.

The vagus nerve

The human digestive tract has around 500 million neurons that communicate with the brain via nerves. The vagus nerve is a major nerve that connects the digestive system to the brain and spinal cord. Negative

effects on the vagus nerve have been linked to psychological stress. Evidence suggests that this may play a
role in the development of inflammatory bowel disease
and irritable bowel syndrome.

Neurotransmitters

Substances called neurotransmitters can communicate
between the central nervous system and the digestive
tract. Some neurotransmitters are synthesized in the
brain and have an effect on emotional regulation, mood
maintenance, and the "fight or flight" response. Their
production can alter gastrointestinal function in the
digestive tract. Studies have demonstrated that neurotransmitters like dopamine, norepinephrine,
epinephrine, and serotonin can affect things like blood
flow, bowel function, nutrient absorption, and the
composition of the microbiome.

How can gut malnutrition affect the brain?

There is a well-established network of nerves and glia
connecting the gut to the brain, and it is from there that
endorphins are produced. They communicate with one
another through a series of messages. For instance,
digestive issues like gas and bloating might make it
difficult to get a good night's rest. However, if your gut
is healthy, it will send signals to your brain that everything is fine there. The vagus nerve, which runs from

the brain to the stomach, has been linked to issues with mental health and vitamin deficiencies. The vagus nerve aids in digestion by stimulating the production of digestive enzymes and sending signals to the brain about satiety (or lack thereof).

The vagus nerve runs from your digestive system all the way up to your brain. The vagus nerve receives signals from the intestines about changes in the microbiota and relays them to the brain during digestion. When the vagus nerve is healthy, the brain instantly responds with the appropriate response. For instance, if you eat anything that causes intestinal inflammation, the vagus nerve will pick up on this and send a message to your brain. Hi, cranium. There's inflammation in this area. Take action!

The brain then relays this signal to the intestines, where a biological mechanism is kicked off to reduce the inflammation. It's like calling in the fire department when your house is on fire. Incredible, huh? If your vagus nerve is damaged or you have a weak vagus nerve, information between your digestive system and your brain will not travel as smoothly. Picture yourself having difficulty receiving calls on your cellphone. You could understand part of it, but you risk missing out on key details. Inflammation is something for which the brain needs to be notified via the vagus nerve in order to "send the fire department." Inflammation worsens and may become persistent in rare circumstances.

The gut-brain axis and mental health

While most focus on the nervous system is on the brain and spinal cord, an equally complex neural system is located in the digestive tract. More nerve cells than the spinal cord can be found in the enteric (or gut) nervous system. When we eat, those nerves are activated. When we start t feel full, our stomach's stretch receptors light up and to the brain.

However, nerves aren't the only factor. The trillions of microorganisms that call our digestive tract home also play a significant role in how our intestines and brains interact. The types of bacteria we carry may impact gut motility, digestive secretions, inflammation, and even neurotransmitter production. Serotonin, also known as the "feel-good" neurotransmitter, is abundant in the gastrointestinal tract. Ninety-five percent of the serotonin in our bodies is produced in the intestines, not the brain.

When we take care of the good bacteria in our digestive tract, they, in turn, send signals to the brain that can have a calming effect. When we're feeling good in our bodies, our brains release feel-good chemicals like serotonin, dopamine, and oxytocin. Mood-boosting hormones are produced in response to food; therefore, our diets directly impact our emotional states. Digestive issues might have a negative impact on short-term brain function. Dysbiosis, or an imbalance of gut microorganisms, can also contribute to inflammation. High amounts of inflammation in the body can have adverse effects on brain function, including memory, emotion, and aggression.

Chronic inflammation is not the only possible element or cause of depression, but it does seem to play a role. Since inflammation is a reaction of the immune system, and since roughly 70% of immune activity occurs in the gut, it stands to reason that when our gut health is less than optimal, our body reacts in several different ways.

In the 'leaky gut' model, poisons and microorganisms enter the bloodstream through minute holes in the gut wall brought about by the inflammatory response. The brain or the immune system could be irritated by these toxins. Beneficial gut bacteria secrete chemicals that feed the blood-brain barrier. Long-term changes in gut health may affect mental well-being since gut function depends on and has consequences for the function of your immune and brain systems.

There is evidence that digestive disorders like IBS and IBD contribute to a higher incidence of emotional distress. They are believed to involve a combination of inflammatory and nervous system effects in the gut and a negative impact on quality of life. People with IBS and depression or anxiety had different microbiomes than those with just IBS, according to research. People with undiagnosed celiac disease may develop brain fog due to the severe inflammation and alterations to the intestinal barrier that occurs during the course of the disease.

More minor mood shifts can also occur as a result of common digestive issues like bloating and constipation. No matter the circumstances, your disposition will suffer if you aren't feeling well or are anxious about your health. Feelings of sluggishness, lethargy, or mental fogginess may accompany temporary alterations in gastrointestinal function.

Let's have a peek at what the next chapter covers:

- Vagus Nerve: The vagus nerve is the primary parasympathetic egress route from the thorax and belly to the cardiovascular and gastrointestinal systems
- Psychological and Inflammatory Disorders Involving the Vagus Nerve's Role as a Modulator of the Brain-Gut Axis
- The Role of the Vagus Nerve in Digestive Wellness

- The Vagus Nerve and Digestion: Eight Connections
- How the gut can Influence the Brain
- How the brain can Influence the Gut
- What Causes Vagus Nerve Dysfunction?
- Vagus Nerve Dysfunction and Its Effect on the Digestive System

3

THE VAGUS NERVE: YOUR BODY'S SECRET MESSENGER LINKING THE BRAIN AND GUT

VAGUS NERVE (VN)

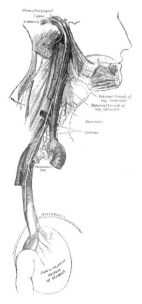

Photo credit: www.physio-pedia.com

Gut and Glory: How the Vagus Nerve Sends Top-Secret Memos Between Your Brain and Belly!

As the "superhighway" of the nervous system, the essential vagus nerve transmits signals from the brain to the rest of the body's organs and controls how the body responds when at rest. Functions of this large nerve, which originate in the brain and runs multiple directions to the neck and torso, including relaying sensations from the ear's skin, controlling the muscles required for swallowing and speaking, and modifying the immune system.

The vagus nerve, or cranial nerve X, is the longest of the mixed cranial nerves. The vagus nerve is a pair of nerves originating in the brain stem's medulla oblongata and is commonly referred to as a single nerve. The vagus, meaning "wanderer" in Latin, connects the cerebral cortex to the brainstem and the hypothalamus, and the rest of digestive system relays information from the body's internal organs to the brain, including the digestive tract, lungs and heart, stomach and intestines, spleen, liver, and kidneys. This nerve plays roles in speech, eye contact, facial expressions, and even the ability to tune in to other people's voices.

It consists of countless strands that work beneath the threshold of our awareness. It's crucial to maintaining good health in general. It plays a vital role in the parasympathetic nervous system, which helps relax muscles and organs following the stressful "fight-or-flight" response.

Functions

The vagus nerve can be found almost anywhere in the body.

- Sensory: This nerve innervates the external acoustic meatus's larynx, throat, and skin. The sensation is brought to the organs in the abdomen and the heart.
- Special Sensory: The epiglottis and the base of the tongue receive taste sensations from this nerve.
- Motor: Motor innervation is provided to most pharyngeal, soft palate, and laryngeal muscles.
- Parasympathetic: Controls heart rate and rhythm through innervating gastrointestinal, respiratory, and gastrointestinal smooth muscles. The cardiac branches lower heart rate, the bronchial branch narrows airways, and the esophageal components regulate the involuntary muscles of the gallbladder, pancreas, esophagus, stomach, and small

intestine to increase peristalsis and gastrointestinal secretions.

Pathway of the Vagus Nerve

From the brain, the vagus nerve travels down through the chest and the abdomen.

- Leaves the brain via the jugular foramen in the skull's side from the brainstem's medulla oblongata.
- The internal jugular vein is located medially to the internal carotid artery and dorsally to the internal carotid artery as it travels down into the sheath.

The vagus nerve splits into the right and left at the base of the neck and follows separate courses through the thorax.

- Beyond the primary right bronchus and esophagus, the right vagus nerve travels into the chest cavity behind the innominate artery and the first section of the subclavian artery, eventually meeting the left vagus nerve in the esophageal plexus.
- After entering the chest between the left common carotid and left subclavian arteries,

the vagus nerve winds its way behind the significant left bronchus.

The vagus nerve is connected to the accessory nerve (CN XI) at the level of the inferior ganglion.

Parasympathetic Actions

The vagus nerve is the primary parasympathetic egress route from the thorax and belly to the cardiovascular and gastrointestinal systems.

1. **The Heart**: The parasympathetic nervous system supplies the heart's sino-atrial and atrioventricular nodes via cardiac branches that originate in the thorax. The activity of these limbs causes the heart rate to slow down at rest. They never stop moving, setting a steady pace of sixty to eighty beats per minute. If the vagus nerve were cut, a person's resting heart rate would drop to about 100 beats per minute.

2. **Gastrointestinal System**: The vagus nerve gives the abdominal organs their parasympathetic nervous system. Up to the splenic flexure of the large colon, this organ supplies the esophagus, the stomach, and most of the intestines. The vagus nerve sends signals to these organs' glands and smooth muscles,

causing them to produce more secretions. For instance, the vagus nerve boosts acid production and accelerates gastric emptying.

GUT-BRAIN AXIS

Our knowledge of the brain-gut axis has undergone a dramatic paradigm shift in the past decade. The brain, stomach, and autonomic nervous system are all connected by a communication network known as the microbiota-gut-brain axis. The vagus nerve (VN) is the primary afferent and efferent nerve in the parasympathetic nervous system, with an afferent (inward towards the central nervous system) fiber content of 80% and an efferent (outward away from the central nervous system) fiber content of 20%. As part of its function in interoception, the VN receives information from the gut via afferents and sends it to the brain, where it is processed and incorporated into the central autonomic network, generating an appropriate reaction.

- The VN's fibers have been linked to a cholinergic anti-inflammatory system that can reduce peripheral inflammation and intestinal permeability, likely altering microbiota composition.

- Stress may play a role in the pathophysiology of inflammatory bowel disease (IBD) and irritable bowel syndrome (IBS) due to its effects on the vagus nerve (VN) and the gastrointestinal tract and microbiota.
- Those with inflammatory bowel disease or irritable bowel syndrome often have a low vagal tone, which promotes inflammation in the body's periphery.
- The growing body of research on the two-way communication between the digestive tract and the brain provides strong backing for a holistic model incorporating the brain's neurological, digestive, and immunological systems.

The vagus nerve has anti-inflammatory effects.

According to heart rate variability, low vagal tone indicates inflammatory bowel diseases and functional digestive disorders. The goal of treatment for such conditions is restoring normal vagal tone. Compared to other therapeutic options like cholinergic-targeting medicines and alternative medicine (deep breathing, hypnosis, meditation, and exercise), VNS (vasomotor nerve stimulation) is a promising new direction. New evidence has recently supported the VNS's function in regulating gastrointestinal functions.

With about 80% afferent and 20% efferent fibers, the vagus nerve (VN) plays multiple critical roles in the homeostatic regulation of visceral functions through communication between the brain and the organs. According to new research, the VN might help reduce inflammation. There are several ways to facilitate this vagal function. The first is the anti-inflammatory hypo-thalamic-pituitary-adrenal (HPA) axis, where vagal afferent fibers activate the adrenal glands and efferent (CAP) fibers secrete cortisol. The autonomic nervous system's vagus nerve (VN) looks to be an excellent ther-apeutic target in inflammatory gastrointestinal diseases (such as IBD) and other inflammatory diseases (such as RA, etc.), given its central involvement in brain-gut interactions.

PSYCHOLOGICAL AND INFLAMMATORY DISORDERS INVOLVING THE VAGUS NERVE'S ROLE AS A MODULATOR OF THE BRAIN-GUT AXIS

The vagus nerve acts as a sensory relay, sending afferent nerve signals "upstream" to the brain from the body's organs. In reality, the vagus nerve has 80–90% of its nerve fibers devoted to relaying information from the internal organs to the brain.

The vagus nerve is the central component of the parasympathetic nervous system, which regulates various vital biological processes (such as mood, immunity, digestion, and heart rate, among others). Through its afferent fibers, it links the brain to the gastrointestinal system and relays information about the health of the internal organs to the brain.

- Vagus nerve stimulation (VNS) has shown early promise as an adjunct treatment for patients with depression, PTSD, and inflammatory bowel disease who have not responded to standard therapies.
- Vagus nerve stimulation and other treatments boost vagal tone and reduce cytokine production. Both contribute significantly to a person's ability to bounce back from adversity. Vagal afferent fiber stimulation has been linked to improvements in major mental diseases like depression and anxiety by affecting monoaminergic (liberating hormones such as serotonin and norepinephrine) brain systems in the brain stem.
- Preliminary research suggests that the bacteria in your gut may positively impact your mood and anxiety levels by modulating vagal nerve activity. Because breathing can change the vagal

tone, which is associated with the ability to regulate stress responses, practices like meditation and yoga are likely to help with resilience and the reduction of mood and anxiety symptoms.

- Various illnesses, including chronic epilepsy, refractory epilepsy, and depression, can now be treated with VNS, thanks to FDA approval. It is also being studied about several other medical issues, such as autoimmune and chronic inflammatory disorders.

Vasovagal Syncope

The vagus nerve contributes to dizziness and fainting caused by heat, prolonged standing, or unexpected stimuli like the sight of blood. Syncope caused by the vasovagal reflex occurs when the sympathetic nervous system dilates blood vessels in the legs, and the vagus nerve overreacts, leading to an abnormally low heart rate. When a person's blood pools in their legs, their blood pressure decreases, and their brain doesn't get enough blood, they temporarily lose consciousness. It is not necessary to treat vasovagal syncope unless it occurs regularly.

THE ROLE OF THE VAGUS NERVE IN DIGESTIVE WELLNESS

Digestion, absorption, and excretion are all governed by how well your vagus nerve functions. So, let's review how improving vagus nerve function aids digestive health. First, remember that the vagus nerve is responsible for 80% of the parasympathetic nervous system in the human body. This is essentially our "sit back and relax" system. The best digestion happens when we're relaxed and at ease. The vagus nerve, whose origins may be traced back to the base of the brain, branches off into the ear and then innervates facial and pharyngeal muscles. It also innervates our digestive system and our hearts' SA (sinoatrial) node. For this reason, the vagus nerve warrants special attention whenever problems with gastrointestinal motility are present. Chronic stress or trauma, for instance, has been linked to decreased stomach motility and enzyme activity, which can lead to digestive problems.

The Vagus Nerve and Digestion: Eight Connections

In the following section, we'll go through all eight of the vagus nerve's roles in digestion.

Regulates the breakdown of solids

The vagus nerve speeds up the digestive process after eating solid foods. Unless you have a medical condition requiring you to eat softer foods, you probably consume solid foods, which is vital. We must be able to digest food before it travels through the complete digestive system. Otherwise, many of us may experience heartburn, bloating, and farting symptoms.

Stimulates the secretion of saliva

The digestive process begins when we put food in our mouths. The salivary glands in our mouths secrete digestive enzymes. The meal is partially digested before it reaches the esophagus.

Promotes the production of gastric acid and bile.

It encourages the production of pancreatic digestion enzymes and liver bile. These play a crucial role in preparing food for transit through the stomach, esophagus, small intestine, and large intestine before being expelled.

Allows the stomach to expand for food.

When the vagal tone is expected, the stomach expands to make room for food. In addition, hydrochloric acid and pepsin help digest the protein in our food even further.

Slows gastric emptying

This is crucial because we want to avoid having the food leave the body too quickly. If the stomach empties slowly, the food's nutrients will be absorbed appropriately.

Coordinates the Motility of Intestines

Nutrient absorption occurs in the small intestine when food reaches that part of the digestive tract. Food is digested once in the large intestine and passed out of the body through the rectum. The vagus nerve plays a crucial role in the small intestine by stimulating the migrating motor complex to produce a wave-like movement that aids food transportation to the large intestine.

Reducing inflammation and gut transparency

Leaky gut is another name for intestinal permeability. The integrity of the tight connections in the gut's epithelial lining is compromised when vagal nerve function, motility, and nutrition assimilation are impaired. This results in the free circulation of pathogens, poisons, undigested food, and bacteria throughout the body, which triggers an inflammatory response from the immune system. Numerous long-term health problems may result from this.

Increase Satiety

You'll be able to tell the difference between being hungry and full if your vagus nerve is healthy and functioning properly. When this is thrown off, and the vagal tone is low, diagnosis can be a challenge. Either you overeat or don't eat enough. Whether your goal is to shed a few pounds or improve your health and athletic performance, this idea is straightforward but crucial. The vagus nerve plays a vital role in digestion. It's giving the gut system its nervous system. Chronic stress, low vagal tone, wrath, anger, worry, anxiety, and the freeze response (frozen while extremely alert, unable to move or take action) are just a few conditions that can seriously harm gut health. Some of those mentioned above have been related to a wide range of gastrointestinal problems. Enhancing vagus nerve function is essential for improving digestive health.

HOW COME THE VAGUS NERVE IS SO CRITICAL?

The vagus nerve's most recognized role is in mediating parasympathetic control of the digestive tract. Connecting the brain to the gut and the gut to the brain acts as a two-way street. The vagus nerve, figuratively represented as a road, constantly transports signals in both directions.

How the gut can Influence the Brain

A "second brain" describes the enteric nervous system (ENS), the neural system of the digestive tract. This is because it coordinates numerous gastrointestinal processes and maintains constant lines of communication with the brain and vagus nerve. To achieve this, we employ:

- Bacteria in the intestines produce chemicals that can operate directly on the brain.
- The immune system, of which 80 percent is located in the gastrointestinal tract and continuously communicates with the central nervous system

How the brain can Influence the Gut

This line of communication between the brain and the digestive system continually relays chemical information designed to enhance the gut's performance. These signals accomplish the following goals:

- Encourage the production of mucus and biofilm in the digestive system; this "slime" of the gut lubricates, moisturizes, and protects the gut lining.

- The surrounding muscles in the digestive system should be stimulated to contract to increase digestive motility.
- Encourage the microbes to produce compounds that promote faster cellular renewal in the digestive system.
- When opportunistic infections reach the digestive tract, they must communicate with the immune system and help regulate it.

WHAT CAUSES VAGUS NERVE DYSFUNCTION?

Severe symptoms or diseases might develop when the gut and vagus nerve link becomes dysfunctional. The vagus nerve acts as a "highway," carrying messages from one part of the body to another. Physical damage to the nerve (such as from a head injury or other trauma) can increase, slow down, or block these neurological impulses. Minor and major concussions (including those caused by fainting or whiplash), chronic stress, gut dysfunction, poor food, disordered breathing, poor oral health, inactivity, and some drugs can all compromise the vagus nerve's health and function.

Vagus Nerve Dysfunction and Its Effect on the Digestive System

Whether the vagus nerve is too active or inactive causes different symptoms. Common side effects of vagus nerve dysfunction include:

Difficulty Swallowing

Damage to the vagus nerve can result in issues with swallowing. Damage to the nerve can also cause problems with the gag reflex. In addition, damage to the vagus nerve can cause changes in your voice since it controls muscles in the throat.

Delayed Gastric Emptying

A sluggish stomach could be the result of damage to or under activity of this nerve. Stimulating the vagus nerve can help control peristalsis, the process by which the muscles of the digestive tract contract and relax to move food along. It has been related to issues like constipation, bacterial overgrowth, feeling full quickly, nausea, heartburn, loss of appetite, stomach discomfort, spasms, and weight loss.

Irritable Bowel Syndrome (IBS)

Irritable Bowel Syndrome (IBS) symptoms include constipation, diarrhea, or both. Abdominal pain or discomfort is a common symptom of IBS. It's also possible that autonomic nervous system dysregulation contributes to irritable bowel syndrome. If the vagus nerve is overactive, this leads to greater stimulation in the digestive system. The subsequent urgency linked with bowel movements, potentially causing abdominal discomfort, might be problematic. Intriguingly, higher blood pressure is also associated with more significant rectal distention, which means that stool has a greater chance of remaining in the rectum for a longer period of time and thus contributing to constipation.

The vagus nerve's tone determines its functionality.

The vagus nerve's tone is crucial in stimulating the parasympathetic nervous system, which helps the body relax and digest food. Vagal tone is assessed by monitoring heart rate in conjunction with respiration rate. A healthy person's heart rate rises with each inhalation and falls with each exhalation. Vagal tone is higher when there is a larger difference between the heart rate on inhalation and exhalation. Increased vagal tone means quicker recovery from stress. However, maintaining vagal nerve tone requires regular exercise, like maintaining muscular tone.

Simple vagus nerve stimulation exercises you can do at home

Exposure to the cold. The vagus nerve becomes active when cold water shuts down the sympathetic nervous system. Turn the water pressure down too low and run cold water over your face as a final rinse. Try a 30-second cold soak followed by a 30-second hot soak to cover your entire body. Two or three 30-second breaks, and then up to 60 seconds.

Diaphragmatic breathing. The average person takes in the air 10–14 times per minute, which indicates shallow breathing. The sweet spot is somewhere around six times per minute. Stress hormones are released by activating the vagus nerve and the parasympathetic nervous system, and the "fight or flight" response is suppressed. Therefore, diaphragmatic breathing is another highly effective vagal stimulation strategy. Here is a helpful method:

1. Put a hand on your stomach.
2. Pull your stomach in as you inhale through your nose. Your tummy will be pushing on your hand, pulling it away.
3. Take a deep breath and count to six before holding it for two counts; then, with a sigh, release the breath completely.

Increased salivation. When the body is in parasympathetic mode, the vagus nerve is stimulated, causing the mouth to produce copious amounts of saliva. This indicates that your body is relaxed and ready to digest meals. If you want to make yourself salivate, sit back in a chair and picture a juicy orange. Allow your mouth to fill with saliva.

Gargle. Repeatedly rinsing your mouth with water (or your saliva) can help prevent bad breath. The vagus nerve stimulates the throat muscles at the back of your mouth, which contract when you gargle. When you gargle, you tighten these muscles, which enables the vagus nerve and, in turn, the digestive system.

And, in turn, the digestive system.

Let's have a peek at what the next chapter covers:

- The microbiota and microbiome of the human digestive tract
- Why is the human microbiome essential?
- The Importance of Your Gut Microbiome to Your Health
- Possible weight changes caused by your gut microbiome
- Possible Heart Benefits from a Healthy Microbiome in the Gut

4

THE GUT MICROBIOTA: AN ECOLOGICAL WONDERLAND INSIDE YOU

Gut Microbiota: Where Trillions of Tiny Guests Make Your Belly Feel like a Happening Party District... Just Don't Ask About the Noise Complaints!

THE MICROBIOTA AND MICROBIOME OF THE HUMAN DIGESTIVE TRACT

The human microbiome is home to trillions of microorganisms, including bacteria. Although most bacteria in the body are beneficial, an imbalance can cause disease. The terms "microbiota" and "microbiome" are commonly used synonymously. But that is not the case. All the different kinds of bacteria, viruses, fungi, and other microorganisms in the human digestive tract, are collectively referred to as the microbiota. The term "microbiome" refers to the collection of microbes, genes, and environmental factors that comprise the human body's natural home.

What is the human microbiome?

Ten to one hundred trillion microbial cells live harmoniously with the human host. Some studies have found that there are as many as ten times as many microbial cells as human cells in the body, while others have found the ratio to be closer to 1:1. As long as the host is healthy, the microorganisms and their host are in a mutually beneficial symbiotic relationship. The human microbiome consists of hundreds of thousands of microbes of various types. Human biome components span a broad spectrum of diversity. There will also be distinct microbial populations in various organs and tissues. Microorganisms can be found in many different parts of the body: the mouth, genitalia, skin, intestines, and lungs. However, the precise types, shades, and characteristics will vary geographically.

What is the gut microbiota?

The vast and intricate collection of bacteria known as the gut microbiota significantly impacts human health. "gut microbiota" has replaced the older term "microflora of the gut." Many body processes rely on the assistance of the gut microbiota, such as:

- Energy extraction from food that has been digested
- Warding against infectious diseases
- Controlling the immunological response
- Increasing the integrity of the gastrointestinal tract's biochemical defenses

These capabilities are vulnerable to shifts in the composition of the microbiota. There are both good and bad bacteria in the digestive tract; the latter can cause infection if they make it past the good guys (good bacteria). Food poisoning and other gastrointestinal illnesses can cause similar symptoms.

WHY IS THE HUMAN MICROBIOME ESSENTIAL?

In many ways, microorganisms are essential to human survival. There may be a connection between the following disorders and the make-up of bacterial populations, as well as the frequency with which disruptions occur:

- Eczema
- Multiple sclerosis
- Obesity
- Heart disease
- Malnutrition
- Asthma
- Autistic spectrum disorder
- Cancer
- Celiac disease
- Diabetes

Nutrition

Microorganisms in the human digestive tract play a vital role in ingesting nutrients and converting them into usable energy. Bacteria in the intestines aid in the digestion of tough foods like meat and vegetables. Cellulose from plants can only be broken down with the help of good bacteria in the gut. Intestinal bacterial metabolic activity has been linked to changes in feeling full or hungry. The diversity of a person's diet can be seen in their gut microbiota.

Immunity

Some researchers have proposed the theory of prenatal exposure to microorganisms. These ancient microorganisms, adaptive immunity would not develop. This central defense mechanism acquires the knowledge necessary to act in response to certain microorganisms. This facilitates a more rapid and comprehensive response to pathogens. The gut microbiota of an individual matures from the time of their initial microbial exposure until they are between three and five years old. Disruptions from these early exposures can hinder the growth of the microbiota.

Behavior

There is continuous two-way communication between a person's gut bacteria and their brain. The gut-brain axis is particularly important for intestinal function. However, there have been connections found between the gut microbiome and mental health issues like depression and autism spectrum disorder.

Disease

Several inflammatory bowel diseases (IBD) have been linked to alterations in the makeup of the gut microbiome, including ulcerative colitis and Crohn's disease. Obesity and type 2 diabetes have been linked to low microbial diversity in the gut. Relationships between the health of the gut microbiota and the metabolic syndrome have been found. Prebiotics, probiotics, and other dietary changes may help lower this risk.

Antibiotic use disrupts the microbiota, which increases the risk of illness and antibiotic-resistant diseases.

Since the "good" bacteria compete with the "bad," and some even secrete anti-inflammatory compounds, the microbiota plays a vital role in preventing the expansion of disease-causing populations introduced from outside the body.

Microbiome research

The genetics of microbial communities in the body and their connections to health and disease have been the subject of massive investments in research. Researchers will be able to classify and analyze the different microbial compositions of the gut microbiota and have a better understanding of their genetic makeup because of this initiative. More recent research confirms that it is possible to introduce a new strain into an established microbiota by exploiting nutrition availability without disrupting the microbiome's natural stability and function. This can pave the way for future probiotic treatments and innovative approaches to understanding gut microbiota composition.

THE IMPORTANCE OF YOUR GUT MICROBIOME TO YOUR HEALTH

The microorganisms and bacteria in your digestive tract aid in food digestion and may also improve your immune system, cardiovascular system, and neurological system. Trillions of microbes (bacteria, viruses, and fungi) live in and on your body. As a group, they are called the microbiome. Some bacteria are linked to illness, but others have major affect system, cardiovascular system, and even how much you weigh.

Bacteria, viruses, fungi, and other forms of life that are only a few microns in size are all considered microorganisms (or "microbes" for short). Millions of these microbes live on and in your skin and digestive tract. The majority of the bacteria and other microorganisms in your digestive system are found in a "pocket" of your large intestine called the cecum, making up what is known as the gut microbiome.

A microbial ecosystem exists within you, with bacteria being the primary research interest. The human body has roughly 30 trillion human cells and 40 trillion bacterial cells. There are up to a thousand different bacterial species in the human gut microbiome, and they all serve crucial roles. Most are necessary for health, but some are dangerous. Five to ten pounds (two to two and a half kg) is a reasonable estimate for the total mass of these microorganisms, which is roughly equivalent to your brain's massive as supplementary organs and are essential to your health.

How does it affect your body?

Over millions of years, mankind has learned to coexist alongside microorganisms. Microbes have evolved to perform crucial functions within the human body during this time. In fact, life without the intestinal microbiota would be quite difficult. Your gut microbiota starts affecting your health as soon as you're born. The birthing process introduces you to bacteria and viruses for the first time. However, recent discoveries indicate that prenatal contact with bacteria may occur. The variety of microbes in your gut microbiome, or "gut flora," increases as you age. A more varied microbiome is thought to have health benefits. It's interesting to note that the foods you eat have an impact in the variety of bacteria in your digestive tract. The expansion of your microbiome has numerous physiological effects, such as:

- **Digesting breast milk:** Bifidobacteria are among the first bacteria to colonize a newborn's intestines. They metabolize the growth-promoting carbohydrates in breast milk.
- **Digesting fiber:** Important for gut health is the short-chain fatty acids produced when some bacteria consume fiber. Getting enough fiber in your diet may reduce your risk of

developing diabetes, heart disease, and even cancer.

- **Helping control your immune system:** Your gut flora also controls how well your immune system functions. Through communication with immune cells, the gut microbiome controls the body's reaction to infection.
- **Helping control brain health:** Recent studies have shown that gut microbiota may also influence the brain and spinal cord.

Therefore, gut microbiota can disrupt vital biological systems and influence health in various ways.

POSSIBLE WEIGHT CHANGES CAUSED BY YOUR GUT MICROBIOME

The vast majority of the hundreds of species of bacteria living in your digestive tract are perfect for you. But an imbalance of good and bad germs might make you sick. Obesity has been associated with gut dysbiosis, in which harmful bacteria outnumber good. Several high-profile studies have demonstrated that the gut microbiota of obese people and their lean counterparts are entirely different. Probiotics, fortunately, promote a balanced microbiota and aid in weight loss. Studies have shown that the average person who takes probiotics loses less than 2.2 pounds (1 kilogram) of weight per year.

It affects gut health.

The microbiome may be a contributing factor in both inflammatory bowel disease (also known as IBD) and irritable bowel syndrome (also known as IBS). Intestinal dysbiosis is a possible cause of the gas, bloating, and stomach pain experienced by people with IBS. The bacteria create gas and other chemicals that might cause intestinal pain. There are harmful microorganisms in the microbiome, but there are also good microbes that promote gut health. Yogurt probiotics like Bifidobacteria and Lactobacillus may help seal off the voids between intestinal cells, preventing leaky gut syndrome. The presence of these species reduces the ability of disease-causing bacteria to attach to the intestinal lining. Consuming probiotics rich in Bifidobacteria and Lactobacilli can help ease the symptoms of irritable bowel syndrome (IBS).

POSSIBLE HEART BENEFITS FROM A HEALTHY MICROBIOME IN THE GUT

Yet another area where the gut microbiota may impact is heart health. In a recent study including 1500 patients, researchers discovered that gut microbiota helped boost "good" HDL cholesterol and triglycerides levels. Some harmful species of gut microbiome species are ese trimethylamine N-oxide (TMAO), which may contribute to cardiovascular disease. TMAO is a molecule linked to atherosclerosis, which can increase the risk of cardiovascular and cerebrovascular disease risk bacteria in the microbiome convert L-carnitine and choline, both of which are present in red r dietary sources derived from animals, into TMAO, which may increase the risk factors for cardiovascular disease. When administered as a probiotic, certain bacteria found in the gut microbiome, particularly lactobacilli, have the potential to lower cholesterol levels.

Aid in glucose regulation and reduce diabetes risk.

The gut microbiome's role in blood sugar regulation may also impact type 1 and type 2 diabetes risk. Thirty-three newborns at high genetic risk for type 1 diabetes were analyzed in a recent study. Researchers discovered that a sharp decline in the microbiome's diversity precedes the development of type 1 diabetes. The study also discovered an increase in the prevalence of certain pathogenic bacterial species preceding the onset of type 1 diabetes. Another study discovered that blood sugar levels could differ substantially even when consumed identical items. The bacteria that live in their digests may be to blame for this.

Affect brain health.

There's some evidence to suggest that the microbiome in your gut is good for your brain, too. To begin, some bacterial species can facilitate neurotransmitter synthesis in the brain. For instance, the antidepressant neurotransmitter serotonin is primarily produced in the digestive tract. Second, millions of nerves run from the intestines to the brain. In this way, the gut microbiota may influence brain health by modulating the transmission of signals along these nerves. Several investigations have demonstrated that the species of bacteria in the intestines of patients with psychiatric problems differ from those of healthy people. The microbiome in your gut affects your brain's health. But it's not clear if this is only because of variations in diet and lifestyle.

How can you boost the microbiome in your gut?

Among the many strategies for fostering a healthier gut microbiome are:

- **Eat a diverse range of foods.** This may result in a more varied microbiome associated with a healthy digestive system. Fruits, vegetables, and legumes, in particular, have a high fiber content that can promote the growth of healthy Bifidobacteria.

- **Eat fermented foods.** The beneficial bacteria found in fermented foods like yogurt, sauerkraut, and kefir, especially lactobacilli, can help lower the population of disease-causing species in the digestive tract.

- **Reduce your use of sugar substitutes.** Some research suggests that aspartame and other artificial sweeteners raise blood sugar by encouraging the growth of bacteria in the gut that aren't good for you, such as Enterobacteriaceae.

- **Eat prebiotic foods.** Prebiotics are a special kind of fiber that helps good bacteria flourish. Foods like asparagus, oats, artichokes, bananas, and apples are all good sources of prebiotics.

- **Do not stop breastfeeding before six months.** Infants' gut microbiomes benefit greatly from breast milk. Breastfed infants have higher levels of beneficial bifidobacteria than bottle-fed infants, and this effect persists for at least six months.

- **Eat whole grains:** Whole grains are a great way to improve metabolic health and reduce the risk of cancer, diabetes, and other diseases since they are high in fiber and beneficial carbs like beta-glucan.

- **Try a plant-based diet:** Switching to a vegetarian diet may reduce cholesterol levels, inflammation, and E. coli and other disease-causing bacteria.
- **Eat foods rich in polyphenols.** Red wine, green tea, olive oil, dark chocolate, and whole grains are all good sources of polyphenols since they contain these plant chemicals. The microbiome degrades them, allowing beneficial bacteria to flourish.
- **Take a probiotic supplement.** When taken after a period of dysbiosis, probiotics can help reestablish healthy gut flora. This is accomplished by "reseeding" the area with beneficial bacteria.
- **Use antibiotics sparingly.** Antibiotics may contribute to antibiotic resistance and weight gain by eliminating both harmful and beneficial bacteria from the gut microbiome. Therefore, antibiotics should be taken only when absolutely essential.

Your stomach is home to a microbiome of bacteria, fungi, and other organisms numbering in the billions. The gut microbiome is essential to health because of the many positive effects it has on the body, including digestion regulation, immune system improvement, and enhancement of other elements of health. The ratio of harmful to beneficial bacteria in the gut is thought to play a role in the development of illnesses such as obesity, diabetes, and high cholesterol. In order to encourage the development of beneficial bacteria in your digestive tract, it's a good idea to eat a wide range of whole grains, fruits, vegetables, and fermented foods.

PART III

YOUR ESSENTIALS GUIDE TO GUT HEALTH

5

A STEP-BY-STEP APPROACH TO HEAL YOUR GUT: REBUILDING HARMONY WITHIN

Gut Rehab 101: When Your Belly Becomes a Construction Zone... Fixing Cracks and Paving the Way for Digestive Serenity!

Having a healthy gut environment is especially important for women over the age of 50. A good gut flora is essential for proper digestion, improving immunity, and mental well-being. The following is a step-by-step strategy to help women over the age of 50 improve their digestive health:

Step 1: Consult with a healthcare professional:

Any significant changes to your diet or way of life should be discussed with your doctor or a competent medical professional, such as a nutritionist or gastroen-terologist. These professionals can tailor their suggestions to meet your individual requirements.

Step 2: Increase dietary fiber:

The importance of fiber in keeping the digestive tract healthy is essential. It's a term for the plant parts our bodies don't absorb and instead flush out. Although they do so differently, soluble and insoluble fiber are essential to gut health.

1. Soluble Fiber: When hydrated, this fiber transforms into a gel. Soluble fiber-rich foods include legumes, oats, barley, apples, oranges, carrots, broccoli, and chia seeds. Soluble fiber aids digestive health in several ways:

2. Soluble fiber serves as a prebiotic, feeding good bacteria in the gut and encouraging their proliferation. These microbes contribute to healthy digestion and create short-chain fatty acids.

3. Soluble fiber prevents constipation because it softens stools by soaking up water and increasing stool bulk.

4. Aids in blood sugar regulation by slowing sugar absorption and reducing the risk of dangerous highs and lows.

5. Insoluble Fiber: This fiber is insoluble in water and helps make bowel movements more substantial. It can be found in the husks of vegetables and fruits, nuts shells, and seeds germination chambers. The following are ways in which insoluble fiber improves digestive health:

6. Constipation is avoided because of the insoluble fiber's ability to add volume to the stool and aid in the transit of waste through the digestive system.

7. Insoluble fiber aids in maintaining a healthy gut pH and feeding beneficial bacteria, both of which contribute to a more balanced microbiome.

A diet rich in fibrous plant foods is advised to promote digestive health. A basic rule of thumb for adults is around 25–38 grams per day of fiber.

Step 3: Stay hydrated:

Keeping yourself well hydrated is crucial to the health of your digestive tract and the healing process. The digestive system dramatically benefits from drinking water.

- Water's lubricating effects on the digestive tract are essential for efficient functioning. Food is moved down the digestive tract with the help of the peristaltic action of the intestines. Maintaining regular bowel motions and good gut motility is facilitated by drinking enough water.

- To absorb nutrients from our food, the digestive tract needs to be well hydrated. Water's ability to carry nutrients past the gut lining and into the bloodstream aids in their absorption.

- The intestinal lining prevents ingested substances from entering the bloodstream. Proper hydration aids in maintaining the intestinal barrier intact by ensuring that the cells lining the intestines remain adequately hydrated. This may improve general gut health and protect against leaky gut syndrome.

- The digestive process and nutrient absorption both benefit from drinking the required amount of water daily. Water is essential for both the digestive process and the disposal of waste. Constipation and other digestive disorders might occur if you don't drink enough water.

- Dehydration is a common cause of constipation. Dehydration makes it more difficult to pass stool because the colon absorbs water from the feces. Constipation can be avoided, and regular bowel movements can be maintained by drinking enough water.

The recommended amount of water to drink each day to maintain hydration and promote healthy gastrointestinal function is eight glasses. Listen to your body's thirst signals to determine how much water it actually needs.

Water isn't the only source of fluids; other meals and liquids can provide them as well. Fruits, vegetables, soups, and herbal teas all fall into this category. Limiting your intake of caffeinated and sugary beverages is recommended for optimal digestive health.

Step 4: Consume prebiotic foods.

Prebiotic meals are highly recommended due to their positive effects on digestion. Dietary fibers called prebiotics may provide beneficial bacteria already residing in your digestive tract. Prebiotics are a class of nutritional supplements that provide food for the beneficial bacteria in the digestive tract. Foods like these, which are rich in prebiotics, are great for anyone seeking to make dietary changes:

- Oats: Prebiotic beta-glucan and other soluble fibers are abundant in oats.
- Apples: Apples are a great source of the prebiotic fiber pectin, which is beneficial to digestion.
- Garlic and Onions: The prebiotic chemical fructans (naturally occurring carbohydrates) are abundant in both onions and garlic. These drugs will increase the number of beneficial bacteria in the digestive tract.
- Legumes: Legumes include diverse foods like peas, beans, and chickpeas. The microorganisms in your digestive tract may benefit from the high fiber content of these foods.
- Flaxseeds: Flaxseeds are an excellent source of fiber and prebiotics.
- Asparagus: Prebiotic fibers like those found in asparagus are crucial to maintaining a healthy gut microbiota.
- Chicory Root: Chicory root has a high inulin content.
- Jerusalem Artichoke: Jerusalem artichokes, or sunchokes, are a fantastic root vegetable source of inulin.

- Bananas: When bananas ripen to perfection, they yield a resistant starch that serves as a prebiotic.

Step 5: Incorporate probiotic-rich foods.

Probiotic-rich meals are beneficial to your gut microbiota and can aid in gut healing. When ingested in sufficient proportions, probiotics—beneficial live bacteria or yeasts—may aid with digestion and strengthen the immune system. Incorporating more of the following probiotic-rich items into your diet may help:

- Tempeh: Fermented soy products like tempeh are packed with healthy bacteria. It's used as a substitute for meat in vegan and vegetarian diets worldwide.
- Kombucha: Natural probiotic bacteria have been discovered in kombucha, a fermented tea drink. It can be enjoyed as a tasty drink and comes in many different flavors. Be wary of pre-packaged foods with a high sugar content.
- Yogurt: Due to its high concentration of probiotic microorganisms, yogurt is frequently consumed. Good options will contain viable probiotic cultures, such as Lactobacillus acidophilus and Bifidobacterium.

- Kefir: Probiotic-rich kefir is a fermented milk beverage. Kefir is a sour and tangy drink created by fermenting milk with kefir grains. Look for yogurts that have live, active cultures.
- Miso: Miso is a Japanese condiment made from fermented soybean paste. It's used to make miso soup and gives other dishes a deep, umami flavor. Find miso that hasn't been pasteurized so you can reap the probiotic advantages.
- Sauerkraut: Sauerkraut, or fermented cabbage, is packed with healthy microorganisms. Find unprocessed sauerkraut if you want to ensure you get all the good bacteria.
- Kimchi: Kimchi, a staple of traditional Korean cuisine, is made by fermenting vegetables like cabbage and radishes with salt and other seasonings. You may enjoy your regular serving of probiotics without sacrificing taste.
- Pickles: Only pickles that have gone through a natural fermentation process (as opposed to vinegar-based pickles) contain probiotics. Look for the terms "raw" or "naturally fermented" on the label to ensure that the pickles you purchase contain live cultures.

Step 6: Reduce processed foods and added sugars.

The digestive system can repair itself and function best when processed foods and added sugars are avoided. Here's how these dietary changes can benefit your gut:

- Decreased Inflammation: The high amounts of refined carbs, unhealthy fats, and chemical additives in processed meals may cause inflammation in the digestive tract and other organs. Over time, intestinal inflammation can kill off beneficial microorganisms that aid digestion.
- Improved Digestive Function: TheStep fiber necessary for effective digestion and regular bowel motions is often missing from processed diets. Eating more complete, fiber-rich meals is one way to aid digestion.
- Reduced Disruption to the Gut Barrier: Processed foods contain common chemicals, artificial sweeteners, and emulsifiers that harm the digestive system. An increased number of toxins can enter the bloodstream when the intestinal barrier is broken. Reduce your risk of developing a leaky gut by cutting back on processed foods.
- Better Blood Sugar Control: Refined carbohydrates, trans fats, and added sugars are

questionable components of processed foods. The sudden rise in blood sugar levels generated by these foods may cause gastrointestinal irritation. A diet rich in whole, natural foods and low in processed foods has been associated with better glycemic management and gastrointestinal health.

- Balanced Gut Microbiome: Most processed foods lack the fiber and other nutrients that foster healthy gut bacteria growth. Fruits, veggies, lentils, and whole grains are all high-fiber foods that may help good bacteria flourish in the digestive tract. Maintain a healthy balance of gut bacteria by eating whole, unprocessed meals and limiting processed food consumption.

Here are some suggestions to help you cut down on processed meals and added sugars:

- Fruits, whole grains, vegetables, legumes, lean meats, and healthy fats should make up the bulk of your diet rather than processed meals.
- Remember to check product labels: Pay attention to food labels and stay away from unhealthy additives like sugar, artificial sweeteners, refined carbohydrates, and bad fats.

- Cooking at home gives you more control over the ingredients and gives you access to less processed, healthier options.
- Limit sugary drinks. Use water, herbal teas, or homemade beverages instead of soda, fruit juice, and energy drinks.
- Reduce your consumption of processed foods by switching to healthy alternatives like fresh fruit, almonds, or homemade granola bars.

Step 7: Manage stress to heal the gut.

Stress reduction is essential for gut health, both during healing and in the long term. Due to the gut-brain axis connecting the two, stress may have a major effect on the digestive tract. The gut microbiome is delicately balanced, and stress may upset that balance, leading to inflammation and digestive problems. Methods to lessen stress and promote intestinal health are listed below:

- Get Adequate Sleep: The consequences of sleep deprivation have been studied and shown to be detrimental in many ways. Create a nighttime routine that allows you to wind down and get the amount of sleep you need each night.
- Social Support: Having a group of friends, relatives, or other people you can talk to and

lean on for emotional support and stress relief may be very beneficial. It has been hypothesized that opening up about how you feel might have beneficial effects on your health.

- Practice relaxation techniques: Some methods of stress reduction include deep breathing exercises, meditating, practicing yoga, and tai chi. These methods have the potential to enhance digestion and gastrointestinal function.

- Regular Exercise: Those who exercise routinely have significant improvements in their stress levels and gastrointestinal health. Exercising regularly is beneficial because it helps keep the microbiota in the gut in good shape. Getting your body moving might be as simple as going for a walk or as complex as learning a new dance move.

- Engage in stress-reducing activities: If you need to relax, go for a walk in the park, put on some calming music, read a book, soak in a hot bath, or meditate. Determine what makes you happy and make it a regular part of your life.

- Time Management: Better time management may lead to less stress and worry. Set priorities and divide up the work. Striking a balance between work, family, and leisure time can help you maintain a healthy weight.

Step 8: Exercise regularly to heal the gut.

The health of your stomach and your body as a whole may benefit from a regular workout routine. Physical activity improves the gut environment and supports digestive function, but it may not cure certain gut disorders on its own. Some of the internal advantages of working out include:

1. Improved digestion: Regular exercise strengthens the muscles of the digestive system, leading to smoother bowel motions and improved digestion. Those who suffer from constipation may find relief from its increased digestive activity.
2. Enhanced gut motility: Regular exercise might help you avoid uncomfortable digestive symptoms like bloating and gas by regulating the rhythm of your stomach contractions. Regular exercise can help balance the gut microbiota and prevent the growth of harmful bacteria.
3. Reduced inflammation: Conditions like IBD and IBS have a common link: they both involve persistent inflammation in the digestive tract.

Exercise may help decrease inflammation everywhere in the body, including the digestive tract.

4. Strengthened immune system: A more robust immune system and a healthy gut microbiome are two benefits of a regular workout routine. Protecting the gut flora balance and warding off infections are benefits of a robust immune system.

5. Stress reduction: Exercise is one of the best ways to reduce stress. Irritable bowel syndrome and other gastrointestinal disorders may develop with high-stress levels. Stress and digestive health both benefit from regular physical exercise.

Step 9: Get enough sleep to heal your gut.

Sleep is essential for good health and may benefit the digestive system. Although sleep does not directly improve digestive health, it is essential in facilitating the body's restorative and healing processes, which include the stomach. Indirectly, sleep might affect digestive health in the following ways:

1. Reducing stress: Stress levels might rise in response to sleep loss or poor-quality sleep. Prolonged stress may significantly impact gut

health by upsetting the usual bacterial balance and causing inflammation. Getting enough shut-eye aids in stress hormone regulation and fosters a more tranquil digestive system.

2. Enhancing immune function: Getting enough sleep each night is crucial for protecting your health. Prevention and treatment of gastrointestinal infections and inflammation require a robust immune system. The production and release of immune cells, antibodies, and other chemicals that promote gut health are facilitated by getting enough sleep.

3. Regulating appetite and metabolism: Sleep deprivation has been linked to abnormalities in the hunger-controlling hormones ghrelin and leptin. These hormonal disruptions may significantly influence gut health by causing an increase in hunger, binge eating, and weight gain. A regular sleeping pattern is associated with less hunger and a more efficient metabolic rate.

4. Supporting the gut-brain axis: The gut-brain axis is a two-way line of communication between the digestive tract and the brain. Adequate sleep helps keep this axis in working order by fostering a favorable microbial balance

in the gut, enhancing gut motility, and decreasing intestinal permeability.

If you want to improve your digestive health through improved sleep, give these tips some thought

- The ideal amount of sleep is seven to nine hours each night.
- Keep a regular schedule for bedtime and waketime.
- Make sure your bedroom is comfortable, quiet, and dark to ensure a restful night's sleep.
- Distracting blue light from phones and tablets at night might be an issue.
- Practicing relaxation methods like deep breathing or meditation may lead to better sleep and fewer nightmares.
- In the hours leading up to bedtime, you should refrain from consuming large meals, caffeine, and alcohol.
- Don't slack off in the afternoon and evening; keep up your regular workout routine.
- See a doctor often if you have difficulties falling or staying asleep.

Step 10: Minimize antibiotic use to heal the gut.

Avoid using antibiotics if you value having a diverse bacterial population in your gut. The hazards of antibiotics, such as damage to the gut flora and stomach troubles, outweigh their benefits in treating bacterial infections. You may need fewer antibiotics to recover from a stomach illness if you follow these steps:

- Only use antibiotics if your doctor says to. Antibiotics cannot be used to treat viral illnesses since they do not work against viruses. Since antibiotics aren't always the most effective treatment for an illness, it's important to explore other options whenever they're available.
- It's possible that taking some probiotics, or "healthy bacteria," can help you get your health back on track. It's important to restore healthy gut flora after taking antibiotics.
- The digestive tract may benefit from a diet high in fermented foods, fiber, and prebiotics (substances that encourage the development of healthy gut bacteria). Eating foods rich in fiber and probiotics has been suggested as a means of maintaining a varied and healthy gut flora, which is essential for efficient digestion.

- If you're experiencing stomach pain or need antibiotics, it's best to contact a doctor. Based on your situation, they may advise, outline the potential advantages and risks of antibiotic treatment, and suggest measures to mitigate gastrointestinal side effects.

Step 11: Eat mindfully to stabilize the gut.

The digestive system benefits from practicing mindful eating. When you eat mindfully, you focus on the process of eating rather than the food itself. Tuning into bodily cues to ascertain fullness is a key component of mindful eating. Just a few of how your digestive system will thank you for paying attention while eating are listed below:

- Mindful eating has been shown to reduce stress levels and is associated with potential improvements in digestive health. Stress, which has been linked to many GI problems, may upset the delicate balance of gut flora. Slow eaters have a better chance of absorbing nutrients from their diet.
- Digestion could benefit from a more deliberate and leisurely eating style. Thoroughly chewed food is easier for the digestive system. Eating more slowly and consciously stimulates the

formation of stomach acid and digestive enzymes, leading to better digestion.

- Mindful eating helps one become more in tune with their own feelings of fullness. The gas and bloating that typically follow a large meal may be avoided if this is kept in mind. It's better for your digestive system if you eat until you're full rather than quitting when you're satisfied.

- Pay close attention to what you eat. Doing so will help your body better process the food and absorb the nutrients it needs. The "food groups" consist of whole grains, vegetables, and fruits. The fiber and good bacteria found in fermented foods like yogurt and sauerkraut have been demonstrated to improve digestive health.

- Evidence suggests that practicing mindfulness while eating might boost nutrient absorption and utilization. Slower eaters may reap the benefits of better digestion and nutritional absorption.

Mindful eating has been linked to sticking to a regular workout schedule. Here are some guidelines to help you get started:

- Refrain from perusing the paper or mail if you're feeling full.

- Take your time and savor every mouthful of your meal.
- Think about your emotional state before, during, and after eating.
- There's more to cooking than simply getting the taste right.
- Evaluate how you feel after eating.

Step 12: Experiment with an elimination diet to heal your gut.

You could try an elimination diet to determine what foods trigger your symptoms. You can gauge your body's reaction to a meal by cutting it out of your diet for a spell and then slowly adding it back in. Read on for an example of an elimination diet.

- Before beginning an elimination diet, it is recommended that you speak with a medical practitioner, such as a registered dietitian or physician, who can advise you on your unique situation and make sure you are getting all the nutrients you need.
- Use the services of a medical practitioner to help you narrow down a list of items that may be triggering your digestive problems. Several foods, such as gluten, dairy, eggs, soy, corn, peanuts, tree nuts, seafood, and some

FODMAPs (fermentable carbohydrates), are known to cause an inflammatory response.

- During the elimination phase, you will refrain from consuming any of the foods that have been determined to be triggers for you. Always check the labels to see if there are any hidden components that could contain the banned foods.

- To keep an eye on your symptoms, keep a food and symptom journal during the elimination period. Keep track of the food you eat and any changes in your health. You'll be able to spot trends and zero in on the offending diet items with this method.

- After the elimination phase is complete, you can begin returning one food type at a time, in modest amounts, while paying great attention to your body's reaction.

- The reintroduction phase. Wait a few days before attempting to eat anything new. To be sensitive or intolerant to a food means to have adverse reactions to it.

- If you pay attention to how your body responds during the reintroduction phase, you'll be able to identify potentially troublesome meals and make necessary adjustments. Not all foods on the list of no-nos will inevitably cause symptoms. Some foods may be safe to eat again, while others may need to be avoided or eaten in moderation.

- A healthcare provider or registered dietitian with expertise in gut health should be consulted at various points along the process for optimal results. They can decipher your signs and symptoms, lead you skillfully through the reintroduction process, and craft an individualized strategy for moving ahead.

Let's have a peek at what the next chapter covers:

- How Fiber Improves Gut Health
- Fiber and the Connection to Gut Health and Your Digestive Tract
- Top 10 High-Fiber Foods
- Implications of Dehydration on Digestive Wellness
- Worst Foods for Digestion
- Probiotics for Gut Health
- Stress can change your gut microbiome
- The gut and sleep
- Proven Tips to Sleep Better at Night

PART IV

YOUR ESSENTIAL GUIDE FOR HEALTHY LIFESTYLE CHANGES THAT SUPPORT GUT HEALTH

6

GASTRONOMIC ADVENTURES: EXPLORING THE WORLD OF GUT-FRIENDLY FIBER, FOODS AND HYDRATION

Gastronomic Adventures: When Your Taste Buds Embark on a Quest for Gutdomination... Join the Gutbusters Guild for Epic Digestive Quests!

This chapter will discuss the steps you need to take to improve your gut health. Let's start with the following:

HOW FIBER IMPROVES GUT HEALTH

Fiber is crucial for overall health because it facilitates elimination, aids in satiety after eating, and keeps the digestive tract in good working order. The gut microbiome relies on prebiotic fiber to function and stay healthy.

Fiber feeds the good bacteria in your gut.

Prebiotics, or plant fibers, can be found in abundance in raw vegetables and fruits. In the large intestine, beneficial bacteria ferment prebiotics for absorption. Protein requirements increase by 5 grams for women beyond age 50. Women should strive for 25 grams of fiber per day.

The intake of enough fiber enhances positive chemical reactions in the body.

Improved immune function and reduced inflammation have both been linked to the short-chain fatty acids and other metabolites produced by the gut flora. The short-chain fatty acids may send a message to your stomach that encourages the growth of healthy bacteria.

Fiber keeps your gut lining intact.

The digestive system acts as a barrier, preventing harmful germs and pathogens from entering the bloodstream while enabling beneficial nutrients to enter. The mucus produced in response to fiber's stimulation of digestive secretions helps reinforce the gut's protective lining.

Fiber balances your gut bacteria.

The microbiome, a collection of bacteria and other microorganisms in the gut, benefits from fiber's ability to maintain diversity. A change in the composition of gut microbes can occur within weeks of starting a high-fiber diet.

TOP 10 HIGH-FIBER FOODS

It may seem difficult to get enough fiber if you aren't in the mood for vegetables. Read on for more delicious, high-fiber food options.

- Beans
- Broccoli
- Berries
- Avocados
- Popcorn
- Whole Grains
- Apples
- Dried Fruits
- Potatoes
- Nuts

How to increase your fiber intake

It's best to acquire your fiber from a wide variety of foods rather than relying too much on any one food group.

You could up your fiber intake by:

- Select a cereal high in dietary fiber, like plain wholewheat biscuits (like Weetabix), plain shredded whole grain (like Shredded Wheat), or opt for porridge made with oats (porridge is another fantastic source of fiber).
- Select wholegrain foods such as granary bread, wholemeal, or white bread with greater fiber content, whole grain pasta, bulgur wheat, or brown rice.
- Choose cooked or boiled new potatoes with the skin on.
- Supplement your stews, curries, and salads with pulses like beans, lentils, and chickpeas.
- Eat a lot of veggies every day, either as a separate side dish or blended into soups, stews, and curries.
- Try some fresh fruit, some dried fruit, or a can of fruit in its own juice for dessert. Dried fruit that is particularly sticky is not good for your teeth and should be eaten only as part of a meal.
- Try rye crackers, oatcakes, unsalted almonds, and seeds, as well as fresh fruit and veggie sticks, as healthy snack options.

Fiber in your daily diet

Here are some common meals, along with how much fiber they contain.

Fiber at breakfast

Two thick slices of whole grain toasted bread (6.6g), one sliced banana (1.4g), and a 150-ml glass of fruit juice (1.2g) add up to around 9.2g of fiber.

Fiber at lunch

Half a can of baked beans (about 200 grams) in low-sugar tomato sauce (9.8 grams) and one baked potato with the skin on (4.7 grams) plus one apple (1.2 grams) equal roughly 15.7 grams of fiber.

Fiber at dinner

9.7g of fiber can be obtained with a diet consisting of a vegetable curry made with tomato, onion, and spices (6.6g), whole grain boiled rice (2.7g), and low-fat fruit yogurt (0.4g). Remember that certain fruit yogurts have a lot of added sugar, so read the label and select the low-sugar options if possible.

Fiber as a snack

Approximately 3.8 g of dietary fiber can be found in a 30-gram serving of nuts like almonds. Choose nuts that aren't salted and have no added sugar.

Fiber on food labels

The quantity of fiber in any given dish will vary depending on factors like how it was prepared and how much of it you ate, so the preceding example should be taken with a grain of salt. Dietary fiber content information is typically included on the nutrition label found on the back or side of most pre-packaged meals.

IMPLICATIONS OF DEHYDRATION ON DIGESTIVE WELLNESS

Getting enough water is crucial to maintaining a healthy digestive system and intestinal tract. Water helps the body distribute nutrients and flush out waste and toxins. But how exactly does water help maintain regular bowel movements, promote healthy skin, and quell inflammation?

Explanation of how maintaining a healthy water intake might benefit the digestive tract.

- Prevents constipation
- Fluids attracted to the digestive tract help move food along in digestion. Symptoms like constipation and bloating can develop if the digestive tract is not supplied with adequate fluid to facilitate the movement of meals.
- Picture yourself sliding down an exciting water slide in a thrilling amusement park. When water can't be used as a propellant, sliding loses

appeal. This is a metaphor like what happens to the stool when the digestive tract dries out.

- Helps break down food for digestion.
- The small intestine uses fluid to carry the acids and enzymes that digest food. It's like a bus that takes the deconstruction team somewhere and then returns with the nutrients.
- Reduces inflammation in the gut
- It's more difficult for food to get through your digestive system when dehydrated. Without adequate fluid transfer, the continual rubbing of food against the intestines can cause inflammation. Inflammation of the intestines might result from this irritant over time.
- Reduces the risk of a permeable gut
- How can intestinal permeability occur? The phrase "leaky gut" has been used to characterize intestinal permeability. This occurs when there is a breakdown in the tight connections in the gut walls.
- This laxity permits poisons, germs, and undigested food particles to enter the bloodstream. Long-term inflammation of the intestinal lining can cause the intestinal walls to weaken and leak. Hydration lowers gut inflammation, which lessens the likelihood of intestinal permeability.

How do you know if you're hydrated?

- You have no sensation of thirst. The human body is remarkably adept at communicating what it requires and when it requires it; we just have to learn to listen. If thirst is your primary sensation, dehydration is likely present.
- You have clear or very light-yellow pee. Urine's golden hue darkens as dehydration progresses. Drink additional water if you see a dark color in your urine.

Five tips to stay hydrated

- Caffeine and alcohol are dehydrating, so cut back as much as possible.
- Have a glass of water first thing in the morning, before each meal, and before bed.
- You may "eat your water" by nibbling on foods like watermelon, strawberries, cantaloupe, celery, and spinach, all of which have high water content. These foods will help you get more fluids because they contain 90 percent water or more.
- Have a water bottle on you at all times. If you keep your water bottle on your desk, you'll be more likely to drink from it regularly.

- Do you dislike the flavor of plain water? Strawberries, lemons, and cucumbers are just a few examples of fresh produce that might go well with this. On hot summer days, frozen blueberries can be added as ice cubes.
- Finally, you know that water is essential for your health, from beautiful skin to a thriving digestive system.

WORST FOODS FOR DIGESTION

Fried Foods

They contain a lot of fat and may cause stomach upset. Even foods like buttery or creamy desserts, fatty meat, and rich sauces should be avoided. Opt for roasted or baked dishes and sauces made with vegetables rather than heavy cream or butter.

Citrus Fruits

Some people may experience stomach distress after consuming them due to their high fiber content and acidity. If you're feeling queasy, it might be best to ease up on the oranges, grapefruits, and other citrus fruits.

Artificial Sugar

Too much chewing of sorbitol-containing sugar-free gum might lead to stomach upset and cramping.

Consumption of foods prepared with this sugar substitute may also harm your health. The FDA advises 50 grams of sorbitol daily, although some people get diarrhea after taking even considerably lower levels.

Too much fiber

Foods rich in this nutrient-dense carb, such as whole grains and vegetables, aid digestion. However, your digestive system may have difficulties adjusting if you suddenly begin eating large quantities of them. This causes intestinal gas and bloating. So gradually increase the amount of fiber in your diet.

Beans

A lack of protein and fiber can have the opposite effect on digestion as eating too many complex carbohydrates. Your body doesn't produce any enzymes that can metabolize them; therefore, they remain unprocessed. Dried beans require at least a four-hour soaking before being used in a recipe.

Cabbage and its cousins

The gas-inducing carbohydrates in beans are also present in cruciferous vegetables like broccoli and cabbage. Because of their high fiber content, they can be difficult to digest. If you boil them before eating them raw, your stomach will thank you.

Fructose

Some people have difficulty digesting foods sweetened with this, such as sodas, candies, fruit juices, and pastries. Consequences may include gas, bloating, and abdominal pain.

Spicy Foods

After a large meal, they can cause indigestion and heartburn in some people. Capsaicin, a component of chili peppers, has been proposed as a possible culprit.

Dairy Products

If consuming them makes you feel ill, you may suffer from lactose intolerance. It indicates a lack of an enzyme necessary for breaking down the sugar found in milk and other dairy products. You can either abstain from eating certain things or take a supplement with the missing enzyme.

Peppermint

Consuming peppermint causes the top stomach muscle to relax, increasing food regurgitation risk. This nearly guarantees you'll experience heartburn.

Losing weight, consuming fewer calories at each meal, and waiting at least an hour before lying down after eating are all recommended by experts to lessen the force pulling on the stomach to urge food back up.

KEEP A FOOD DIARY.

We'd all like to monitor our dietary intake and its effects on our health occasionally. A food diary is the best tool for anyone looking to lose weight, keep track of their calorie consumption, or identify foods that should avoid.

What is a food diary?

When you keep a food diary, you write down everything you consume daily. The app monitors mealtimes, calorie intake, and nutrient balance. Like a food journal, it logs everything you put into your body. A food diary contains all the information you need to evaluate your diet.

Food diary entries to keep track of

These are some of the typical entries found in a food journal.

- What is consumed
- The amount of food consumed
- The timing of meals
- The dining establishment

- Emotional state during mealtime

PROBIOTICS FOR GUT HEALTH

Probiotics are good bacteria that can colonize your intestines. These are the "good" bacteria that research has shown to promote digestive health. Probiotics have gained popularity in recent years as a strategy for better intestinal health and for a good reason. Here I'll discuss the beneficial effects of probiotics on the digestive tract.

Improving Digestive Health

By balancing out the harmful and good bacteria in the digestive tract, probiotics aid with digestion and regular bowel movements. Intestinal discomforts such as gas, constipation, and diarrhea may find relief from this. In addition to improving digestive health, probiotics help lower inflammation in the stomach.

Boosting Immunity

Beneficial microorganisms included in probiotics aid in maintaining immune cells in the digestive tract. In addition to improving immunity, probiotics prevent infections by stunting the growth of harmful bacteria in the gut.

Reducing Inflammation

Chronic disorders such as inflammatory bowel disease (IBD) and autoimmune diseases have been related to intestinal inflammation. Reducing inflammation in the stomach with probiotics can alleviate symptoms and prevent the development of certain conditions.

Improving Mental Health

Probiotics have been linked to better mental health, and studies demonstrate a link between the gut and the brain. Neurotransmitters like serotonin and GABA play a crucial role in mood regulation, and probiotics aid in their production.

Supporting weight loss

Boosting the population of beneficial gut bacteria is one way probiotics can facilitate weight loss. Improved insulin sensitivity and decreased cravings are potential benefits of having these bacteria in the stomach.

Choosing Probiotics

Supplements, fermented foods, and beverages are all good sources of probiotics. When shopping for a probiotic, look for a high-quality supplement with multiple bacterial strains. Probiotics can also be found in fermented foods such as kimchi, sauerkraut, and kefir.

7

CULTIVATING A HARMONIOUS GUT: TRANSFORMATIVE LIFESTYLE SHIFTS FOR GUT-FRIENDLY LIVING

MANAGE YOUR STRESS

Stress can change your gut microbiome.

Stress clearly has a direct relationship to poor gut health since it alters the stomach's normal function and the gut microbiome's composition. Studies have shown that infants born to mothers who experienced high high-stress during pregnancy had reduced quantities of helpful bacteria in their gut microbiomes.

Hormones released in response to stress can significantly enhance the pathogenicity of bacteria and viruses.

Hormones and substances secreted during stress may encourage the growth of pathogenic microbes in the digestive tract. Hormones and substances like catecholamines and serotonin operate as quorum-sensing molecules that can change the virulence of certain bacteria.

Stress messes with your digestive system.

Stress can result in irritable bowel syndrome, acid reflux, SIBO, constipation, diarrhea, and delayed stomach emptying. Common symptoms include constipation, diarrhea, bacterial overgrowth, IBS, delayed stomach emptying, and acid reflux.

EFFECTIVE STRESS RELIEF STRATEGIES

That's why it's so important always to have a supply of stress-relieving activities on hand. Then you can choose the most appropriate tactic for your current situation. Deep breathing and meditation are only two examples of the many effective practices that may be practiced anywhere, at any time. Practice any of the following:

Try guided imagery

In guided imagery, sometimes known as "happy place" meditation, you can imagine yourself in a positive mental state. You can use a recording or just close your eyes and imagine yourself in a tranquil setting to achieve this. Close your eyes, then open them again to return to the here and now.

Meditate

Stress, both immediate and chronic, can be mitigated through meditation. Practicing mantra or mindfulness requires tuning into your senses and focusing on what you perceive. Although it may take some time to master, it has the potential to significantly reduce stress.

Practice progressive muscle relaxation

The goal of progressive muscle relaxation is to gradually loosen every muscle in your body. To train, take a few deep breaths while you progressively tense and release your muscles from your head to your toes. You should feel more at ease after each practice session.

Focus on breathing

You can significantly reduce your stress levels by paying attention to or modifying your breathing patterns. There are a wide variety of breathing exercises available; however, some of the most basic are:

- Feel your stomach expand as you inhale through your nose. While breathing in, try counting to three. For the following three counts, hold your breath for a full second before releasing it through your nose.
- Close your eyes and take a few deep breaths, picturing yourself taking in a wave of tranquility as you do so. Visualize the breeze permeating every inch of your body. Think of your exhalation as releasing tension and anxiety.

Take a walk

The stress-relieving effects of exercise can be felt almost immediately. A walk provides the health advantages of exercise and the mental benefits of a change of scenery. Walking is excellent for the mind and body, whether it's a quick walk around the office to clear your head during a stressful meeting or a leisurely stroll in the park after work.

Get a hug from a loved one

The hormone oxytocin, released during a warm embrace, has been linked to improved mood and reduced stress. In addition to relieving stress, it lowers blood pressure and norepinephrine levels. Don't be shy about asking for comfort in the form of a hug.

Enjoy Aromatherapy

Studies on the effects of aromatherapy on relieving stress have indicated that it increases feelings of vitality, calm, and concentration. A person's emotional response to an odor may influence brain wave activity and alleviate stress. You might incorporate aromatherapy into your regular routine by using candles, diffusers, or body products.

Create Artwork

The meditative act of coloring in a coloring book can reduce anxiety and stress levels. Complex geometric patterns have been demonstrated to alleviate anxiety, making them excellent stress relievers.

Eat a balanced diet

Emotional eating and high-fat, high-sugar foods provide short-term respite, but poor diets might increase responsiveness to stress. High blood sugar from eating refined carbohydrates has been linked to increased stress and anxiety. Eating healthful foods like eggs, avocados, and walnuts can help with long-term stress management.

Supplements for stress relief

The following supplements have shown promise for reducing stress:

- **Melatonin**: The circadian rhythm can be maintained with this hormone. Getting better sleep might help reduce feelings of anxiety.
- **Ashwagandha**: The adaptogenic properties of this plant are supposed to make the body more resistant to mental and physical stress.
- **L-theanine**: This amino acid has been proven to have calming and sleep-inducing effects.
- **B vitamins**: B vitamins have been linked to reduced homocysteine levels, lessened stress, and enhanced mood.

Make time for leisure activities

Engaging in enjoyable activities can be a fantastic way to reduce anxiety and boost productivity. Including time for fun in your calendar can boost your mood and productivity, allowing you to get more done in less time. Hobbies and free time are essential for flourishing.

Develop a positive self-talk habit

It's crucial to have more realistic, caring conversations with yourself. You can respond to negative self-talk with a more encouraging internal monologue. Changing your mindset and taking constructive action are both aided by positive self-talk.

Practice Yoga

Yoga's stress-reducing effects stem from a combination of the practice's physical postures (asana), breathing techniques (pranayama), mental concentration (meditation), and light physical exertion (light stretches). Even though you may get some short-term benefits from a yoga session, consistent practice is what will make a lasting difference in how you feel. Yoga is beneficial for one's physical health, mental well-being, and spiritual growth. We will discuss more on the benefits of yoga.

Express Gratitude

Practicing gratitude is a healthy way to take stock of our blessings and be reminded of our coping mechanisms in times of adversity. Happiness, stress levels, and overall health all improve for the appreciative. Keeping a gratitude diary and writing down at least three things for which we are thankful every day is an important step in making thankfulness a habit.

Prioritize Exercise

Regular exercise is a great way to reduce stress and boost your mood. Numerous options exist, from enrolling at a fitness center or group class to working out in the great outdoors. Exercises like walking, kayaking, hiking, weightlifting, and spin class are just a few examples.

Get enough sleep

Poor sleepers have been found to have less than optimal gut flora and a lower degree of cognitive flexibility. Problems with interruptions to sleep may also hurt the gut microbiome. Heart disease, obesity, diabetes, and depression are just some of the dysbiosis-related chronic illnesses that have been linked to a lack of sleep.

What's going on?

The brain's numerous neurons enable it to communicate with other organs, such as the stomach. The vagus nerve connects the digestive system to the brain and is a part of the gut-brain axis. Intestinal neurons communicate with the central nervous system via neurotransmitters produced by gut bacteria. Such neurotransmitters include GABA, dopamine, and serotonin.

But how does this pertain to sleep?

The pineal gland, which regulates the body's circadian cycle, secretes melatonin, the hormone responsible for inducing sleep. When the pineal gland isn't doing its job, the body falls back on the intestines. Getting a good night's sleep depends on the gut's health because tryptophan is converted to melatonin there.

PROVEN TIPS TO SLEEP BETTER AT NIGHT

Work stress, family obligations, and even physical disease can all disrupt your sleep schedule. Understandably, sound sleep can be hard to come by occasionally. The things that prevent you from sleeping can be beyond your control. You may, however, train yourself to fall asleep more easily. This is the basic starting point.

During the day, expose yourself to more bright light.

The circadian rhythm is your body's 24-hour biological clock and regulates mood, energy, and hormone production. Increased daytime alertness, better sleep quality, and a healthy circadian rhythm are all benefits of exposure to sunlight and other bright light sources at various times of the day. Insomnia patients benefited from daily exposure to bright light by sleeping better and longer and waking up feeling rejuvenated. People who sleep usually can benefit from daily exposure to light.

Cut back on your evening blue-light exposure.

Daytime light exposure is helpful, but nighttime light exposure has the opposite impact because it disrupts the circadian rhythm, decreasing melatonin and other hormones. Particularly harmful is the blue light that electronic devices emit. There are ways to lessen the effects of blue light at night. Among these are:

- Put on some blue-light-preventing glasses.
- Use a blue-light blocking program, such as f.lux, on your computer.
- You should get a blue-light-blocking app for your phone. They work with both iOS and Android devices.
- Two hours before bedtime, switch off all electronics and dim the lights.

Avoid having coffee after 2 p.m.

Due to its many benefits, 90% of people in the United States consume caffeine. However, it can prevent the body from properly winding down at night if ingested late in the day, stimulating the neurological system instead. If you're sensitive to caffeine or have difficulties sleeping, it's best to avoid drinking coffee after 3 or 4 p.m. If you must drink coffee, drink decaf.

Take fewer or shorter naps during the day.

Short power naps are helpful, but napping for too long or too frequently might disrupt nighttime sleep. Those who are accustomed to napping during the day have been proven to have better sleep quality and fewer sleep disruptions at night. Those who aren't accustomed to midday naps are more likely to suffer from poor sleep quality. Naps have variable effects on different people.

Don't tinker with when you plan to be up and asleep.

The 24-hour cycle of light and dark controls the circadian rhythm, also called the biological clock. The quality of your sleep might be enhanced by sticking to a regular nighttime regimen. Alterations to the circadian rhythm and melatonin levels, which signal sleepiness to the brain, can result from not sticking to a normal sleep schedule. Consistently rising and retiring at the same times each day is associated with health benefits.

Take a melatonin supplement.

Studies have revealed that the hormone melatonin can shorten the time it takes to nod out. Studies have indicated that taking 2 milligrams of melatonin before bed will improve sleep quality and make you feel rejuvenated the next morning. Adjusting to a new time zone is another benefit. Before using, check with your physician.

Consider these other stress-reducing supplements

Several supplements can aid in relaxation and sleep, such as:

- **Ginkgo biloba** is a natural plant with multiple uses; some data suggest it helps with sleeping, chilling out, and relieving tension. Just before going to sleep, take 250 mg.
- **Glycine:** Taking 3 grams of the amino acid glycine before bed has improved sleep quality.
- **Valerian root:** Multiple studies have shown that valerian can increase the quality and duration of one's sleep. Take 500mg at night.
- **Magnesium:** Magnesium, involved in over 600 biochemical events in the human body, has been shown to promote calmness and better sleep.
- **L-theanine:** L-theanine, an amino acid, has been shown to facilitate restful sleep. Just before bed, take 100–200 mg.
- **Lavender:** Lavender, a potent herb with many health benefits, is often used to promote relaxation and sleep. Take 25–46% linalool, or 80–160 mg.

Be sure to give each supplement a trial separately. They aren't a panacea, but they can help when used in conjunction with other natural sleep aids.

Don't drink alcohol.

Alcohol consumption in the evening may cause or exacerbate sleep apnea, snoring, and other sleep disturbances. It also affects the circadian rhythm by changing the amount of the hormone melatonin produced at night.

Optimize your bedroom environment.

The design and arrangement of your bedroom can have a significant impact on how well you sleep. Poor sleep and long-term health problems have been linked to environmental noise. Reduce the amount of noise, natural light, and artificial light entering your bedroom for maximum comfort. Make sure your bedroom is a calm, tidy, and pleasant place to spend time.

Set your bedroom temperature.

There is a strong correlation between the temperature of the body and the temperature of the bedroom. Hotter bodies and rooms have been linked to less restful sleep and more time spent awake. Most people, depending on their own tastes and routines, prefer an ambient temperature of about 70 degrees Fahrenheit (20 degrees Celsius).

Don't eat late in the evening.

What you eat late at night may have an effect on how well you sleep, how much growth hormone you secrete, and how much melatonin you make. While having a high-carb meal four hours before bedtime may help you nod off faster, consuming fewer carbohydrates throughout the day has been linked to greater sleep quality.

Unwind and get some mental space before bed.

Insomnia can be alleviated, and sleep quality improved by practicing relaxation before bed. Find out what works best for you by experimenting with various approaches.

Take a relaxing bath or shower.

Bathing or showering before bed can aid in winding down and falling asleep. Taking a hot bath 90 minutes before bedtime has been shown in research to improve both the depth and quality of sleep. Soaking your feet in warm water before bed might help you relax and prepare for sleep.

Rule out a sleep disorder.

Clinically diagnosed sleep disorders include periodic limb movement disorder, obstructive sleep apnea, and circadian rhythm sleep/wake disorder. It's estimated that 9% of women have sleep apnea. If you've had trouble sleeping, you should see a doctor.

Invest in a soft mattress and pillow.

It has been shown that getting a new mattress can decrease shoulder discomfort by 60%, back pain by 57%, and back stiffness by 59%. Lower back pain might be exacerbated by sleeping on poor-quality bedding. Bedding should be replaced every 5–8 years; if you haven't done so in that time, it's time to do so.

Regular exercise is essential, but not right before you turn in for the night.

Regular exercise has been demonstrated to benefit sleep quality as well as overall health. There is potential to increase sleep duration on average by 18%, lessen insomnia symptoms by 15%, and cut back on anxiety and total nightly awake time by 15%. The stimulating effect of exercise, which raises awareness and releases chemicals like epinephrine and adrenaline, may prevent sleep if it is performed too late in the day.

Don't drink any liquids before bed.

Nocturia is the medical name for urinating at night, especially if it wakes you up and makes you tired. Similar symptoms can be brought on by drinking a lot of fluids before bed, so it's best to avoid doing either until after you've used the restroom.

Take Digestive Enzymes

Digestive enzymes hold a key to unlocking optimal gut health for women over 50. As we age, our bodies undergo various changes, including a natural decline in enzyme production. This decline can hinder our digestive processes, leading to discomfort, bloating, and nutrient deficiencies. Incorporating digestive enzymes into our daily regimen can help compensate for this decline and support efficient digestion. These enzymes act as catalysts, breaking down complex nutrients into more easily absorbable forms, promoting nutrient uptake and overall digestive well-being. By supplementing with digestive enzymes, women over 50 can enhance their body's ability to extract vital nutrients from food, alleviate digestive discomfort, and maintain vibrant health as they embrace the transformative years ahead.

Enzymes secreted by the digestive system are necessary for the digestion of food. These proteins aid in the biochemical processes required to transform dietary nutrients into usable forms. The digestion enzymes in saliva are quite helpful. In addition to the pancreas, the gallbladder and liver also manufacture them. The gut mucosal lining cells also store these chemicals.

Catalytic proteins, or enzymes, are proteins that can break down other substances.

- **Amylase** breaks down starches and carbs.
- **Protease** works on proteins.
- **Lipase** handles fats.

Where to Find Digestive Enzymes in Nature

Natural digestive enzymes can be found in foods like fruits and vegetables. Digestive health can be enhanced by eating them.

- Amylase and protease are present in honey, particularly in raw honey.
- The presence of amylase in mangoes and bananas contributes to the ripening process.
- Papain, a protease found in papaya, is an enzyme.
- Avocados are rich in the digestive enzyme lipase.
- During fermentation, sauerkraut, or fermented cabbage, absorbs digestion enzymes.

You won't be able to break down your meal properly if your body isn't producing enough digestive enzymes. That can cause uncomfortable side effects like nausea, vomiting, and gas.

Let's have a peek at what the next chapter covers:

- Top Probiotic Foods
- Foods high in prebiotics promote digestion
- Top Leaky Gut Supplements
- Foods to avoid for a healthy gut
- Effects of Alcohol on the Digestive System
- Antibiotics and the microbiome: a double-edged sword

8

SUPPLEMENTS-PROBIOTICS, PREBIOTICS, AND OTHER GUT FRIENDLY SUPPLEMENTS

Move Over, Picasso: How Gut-Friendly Supplements Turn Your Stomach into a Masterpiece. Bon Appétit-tite

WHAT ARE PROBIOTICS?

The gut microbiome, which contains probiotics, is crucial to health and disease status. Negative consequences can manifest in diarrhea, acne, yeast infections, autoimmunity, and recurrent colds and flu if treatment is inadequate. Due to harmful farming methods and poor nutritional quality, today's food supply contains significantly fewer probiotics. Several probiotic foods can be consumed to aid in providing these vital microbes. The following health benefits may be attained by consuming more probiotic foods:

- Reduced cold and flu
- An increase in energy.
- Probiotics kill candida
- Stronger immune system
- Improved digestion
- Better skin health, as probiotics alleviate skin conditions, including eczema and psoriasis.
- Recovering from IBD and intestinal permeability
- Weight management

TOP PROBIOTIC FOODS

The principal sources of this helpful bacteria are listed below.

Kefir

This unique fermented dairy product is made with milk and kefir grains. It contains anything from 10 to 34 different strains of probiotics and has a somewhat acidic and sour taste. However, since it's lower in lactose and richer in probiotics, it's a good option for those who have lactose intolerance.

Sauerkraut

Sauerkraut, made from fermented cabbage and other probiotic vegetables, has few probiotic strains but is rich in sour-tasting organic acids. It contains a lot of vitamin C and enzymes to aid digestion. It's also rich in lactobacillus and other naturally occurring lactic acid bacteria.

Kombucha

Kombucha is a carbonated beverage that ferments black tea with a symbiotic colony of bacteria and yeast (SCOBY). The critical health advantages of kombucha include supporting digestion, boosting energy, and cleansing the liver.

Coconut kefir

This variant, fermented from young coconut juice using kefir grains, shares some probiotics with traditional kefir but is often lower in probiotic content. However, it does contain some strains that are good for your health. Delicious drinks can be made by combining coconut kefir with stevia, water, and lime juice.

Natto

Natto is a well-liked Japanese dish widely regarded as one of the best probiotic foods due to its high concentrations of the potent Bacillus subtilis and the anti-inflammatory enzyme nattokinase (It can be purchased as a supplement). In addition, it has been shown to improve immunological function, promote cardiovascular health, and reduce the risk of blood clots because of its high protein content.

Yogurt

Greek yogurt, made from the milk of cows, goats, or sheep, is one of the most popular probiotic foods. Yogurt made from grass-fed cows and not pasteurized can be among the best probiotic meals. The issue is that the quality of yogurt available nowadays varies widely. Go for goat's or sheep's yogurt prepared from organic, grass-fed goat's or sheep's milk if you're in the market for yogurt.

Kvass

Fermented beverages containing this potent component have been consumed in Eastern Europe for millennia. Fermented rye or barley was the traditional base, although, in recent years, probiotic fruits and beets have also been used, as have other root vegetables, including carrots. Kvass is a fermented beverage with a mild sour taste and a reputation for purifying the blood and liver, thanks to Lactobacillus probiotics.

Raw Cheese

Probiotics such as thermophiles, bifudus, bulgaricus, and acidophilus are abundant in sheep, goats, and A2 cow's soft cheeses. However, to get probiotics, you must stick to buying raw and unpasteurized cheeses because pasteurized and processed cheeses have been stripped of their helpful bacteria.

Apple cider vinegar

Apple cider vinegar can help increase probiotic intake and its other health benefits, including lowering blood pressure and cholesterol, facilitating weight loss, and promoting insulin sensitivity. Maximize the effects by drinking a little daily or using it as a salad dressing.

Salted gherkin pickles

These delectable fermented snacks are also an underappreciated source of probiotics. If you're in the market for pickles, go for a local, artisanal producer who prioritizes using organic ingredients. Likewise, the best probiotics for your health can be found at a local maker.

Brine-cured olives

Brine-cured olives are a great way to get your daily dose of probiotics. For example, if you're going to buy salted gherkin pickles, choose an organic brand first.

Next, make sure a major producer doesn't create your olives and instead opt for one of the many smaller brands that actively promote the health benefits of probiotics. Olives are a probiotic power food, but if they contain the food ingredient sodium benzoate, they lose some of their health benefits.

Tempeh

This fermented soy product from Indonesia is a great additional source of probiotics. Soybeans are fermented into tempeh by mixing them with a tempeh starter. After sitting for a day or two, the product takes on the consistency of cake. Tempeh is a versatile food that may be eaten both raw and cooked. It can be cooked in the oven, on the grill, in a marinade, or in a skillet to replace meat in a variety of dishes.

Miso

Miso, a staple of Japanese cuisine and medicine, is a traditional Japanese seasoning. It's simple to make by fermenting soybeans, barley, or brown rice with the fungus koji. It's a great spread for crackers, a substitute for butter, and a tasty addition to marinades and stir-fries.

Traditional Buttermilk

The liquid that remains after butter has been churned can be used to make a fermented beverage known as traditional or cultured buttermilk. Remember that most buttermilks you'll get in the supermarket don't have any probiotics. Instead, pick a type that boasts added health advantages from live cultures.

Water kefir

Water kefir, made by fermenting grains in sugar water, is a probiotic-rich carbonated drink. The water variety is highly recommended as a natural vegan probiotic meal to incorporate into a balanced plant-based diet. It's more ethereal than the standard form and can be flavored with various fruits, herbs, and spices.

Raw Milk

Probiotic content is highest in aged cheeses like A2, raw sheep's, goat's, and cow's milk. Remember that probiotics can only be obtained by consuming high-quality, raw dairy that has not been processed; all pasteurized dairy is devoid beneficial enzymes to process.

Kimchi

Similar to sauerkraut, kimchi is a Korean dish made from fermented cabbage. Chinese cabbage, radishes, carrots, ginger, onion, garlic, sea salt, fish sauce, and other ingredients are combined with other ingredients to form this dish. The mixture is then set aside to ferment for three to fourteen days, yielding a savory, probiotic-rich component.

FOODS HIGH IN PREBIOTICS PROMOTE DIGESTION.

Prebiotics?

Both prebiotics and probiotics have been linked to improved health and a more stable microbiome in the digestive tract. Fermented foods like kefir and yogurt contain live microorganisms called probiotics that aid digestion, while prebiotics are indigestible substances that nourish good gut bacteria. Eating a diversified and balanced diet with a range of fruits and vegetables, whole grains, and other fiber-rich foods will assist in developing improved digestive health and overall wellness.

Mushrooms

Carbohydrates such as chitin, beta and alpha glucans, and other substances that function as prebiotics are abundant in most edible mushroom types. Mushrooms are a great source of prebiotics and vital amino acids and minerals like calcium, magnesium, potassium, iron, and zinc, which all help maintain our body's energy levels and defense mechanisms.

Asparagus

Because it can be quickly roasted or sautéed with other vegetables, asparagus is a tremendous non-starchy vegetable to include in your weekly meal prep. Inulin is a soluble dietary fiber found in many foods high in prebiotics; it encourages the growth of good bacteria in the digestive tract. Bifidobacteria have been proven to aid digestion, influence the immune system, and restore the stomach's microbiota after antibiotic treatment.

Seaweed

Due to its numerous health benefits, seaweed is quickly gaining favor in Western diets. There is good vitamin content (A, B1, B12, C, and E) and some insoluble fiber. Some examples of edible seaweed are as follows:

- Hijiki
- Umibudo
- Wakame
- Kombu
- Nori
- Kelp

Jerusalem Artichokes

Jerusalem artichokes are a type of sunflower that grows in the central United States and Canada. Prebiotic substances like inulin , oligofructose, and minerals like potassium can be found in these foods. As a result, they promote healthy bacteria growth and increase mineral absorption, both of which contribute to maintaining a healthy gastrointestinal tract.

Chickpeas, lentils, and kidney beans

Protein, prebiotic carbs, and minerals abound in legumes, making them a smart choice for maintaining digestive and immune system wellness. Intestinal motility, mineral absorption, and obesity risk can all be improved by eating more legumes, which are rich in prebiotic carbohydrates.

Chicory Root

Chicory is a perennial plant with brilliant blue flowers that is a member of the daisy and sunflower families. Because of its abundance, inulin (a prebiotic ingredient) is frequently used as a coffee replacement or fiber addition. Minerals, including potassium, calcium, magnesium, selenium, and zinc, are also present.

Onions, leeks, garlic, and spring garlic

Prebiotic components like flavonoids have been found to positively influence our gut microbiota and enhance immune function and metabolism. The Allium family of vegetables includes onions, leeks, garlic, and spring onions.

Nectarines, watermelon, and blueberries

Carotenoids, fiber, potassium, and antioxidants can all be obtained from fruits in a calorie-efficient manner. The prebiotic chemicals and insoluble fiber in pears, watermelons, blueberries, and nectarines aid digestion.

Oats and barley

The largest concentrations of the prebiotic beta-glucan are found in oats and barley. Beta-glucan, found in high concentrations in whole grains, has been shown to promote the growth of good bacteria in the gut and reduce blood levels of LDL cholesterol and triglycerides.

Dandelion Greens

Dandelion greens have a sour and bitter flavor but are rarely used. Minerals and vitamins like phosphorus, calcium, magnesium, vitamin C, and vitamin K can be found in them.

Cocoa Powder

While chocolate does have some health benefits, eating too much of it can cause you to gain weight and have high blood sugar. Cocoa's antioxidant and probiotic properties make it an effective tool against oxidative stress.

Jicama Root

This Mexican tuber root may have slipped your attention a few times in the supermarket. This tasty root vegetable is crispy on the outside and white and fluffy on the inside, much like eating an apple. As a source of prebiotic inulin, jicama is a fantastic low-carb food choice.

TOP LEAKY GUT SUPPLEMENTS

Proteins like gluten, toxins, and bacteria that aren't digested can leak through the intestinal lining and into the bloodstream in people with leaky gut syndrome. This may trigger an immunological response and systemic inflammation. Food sensitivities, inflammatory bowel disease, arthritis, hypothyroidism, adrenal exhaustion, skin problems, depression, anxiety, nutritional malabsorption, ADHD, and autoimmune diseases can all develop over time if the condition is not treated. Taking the proper nutrients can help heal a leaky gut.

Probiotics

It is crucial for gut health, especially for people with leaky gut, to take a high-quality probiotic supplement. Choose strains carefully to maximize the benefits of the plant's natural medicinal properties. Consider the CFU count, genus, species, and stress while shopping for a probiotic supplement.

Recommended Daily Intake: It is advised that most people take two to four high-quality probiotic capsules daily. In addition to other gut-supporting substances, probiotics may be included in a formulation for leaky gut. Examples of other gut-supporting substances include

- Digestive enzymes
- Prebiotics
- GI Detox
- Betaine Hydrochloride (HCL)

Fiber

Sprouted chia seeds, flaxseeds, and hemp seeds are examples of high-fiber foods that can help foster the development of gut bacteria. If you suffer from a leaky gut, you may need to boil your produce before eating it. In addition, you should consume 30–40 grams of fiber daily if your digestive system isn't susceptible.

Enzymes

You may help your body break down proteins, complex carbohydrates, and carbs by taking digestive enzyme supplements before and after meals. I suggest taking a supplement that offers a wide variety of enzymes, including:

- Lipase: Fat-digesting enzyme
- Lactase: Milk sugar (lactose) is easily digested thanks to lactase.
- Protease: Protease is an enzyme that digests proteins.
- Amylase: Starch-digesting enzyme

In addition, particular enzymes aid the body in digesting various foods. You might ask for a special formula if you have specific dietary requirements, like avoiding gluten or dairy.

L-Glutamine

L-glutamine is an essential amino acid that helps rebuild the lining of the digestive tract and reduces inflammation. The intestinal lining cells rely on glutamine for energy, so it's no surprise that this amino acid is useful for mending a leaky gut. Further, L-glutamine supplementation is warranted since stress depletes glutamine levels, making one susceptible to a leaky gut.

Licorice Root

The licorice root is an adaptogenic plant that helps the body's natural processes preserve the stomach and duodenal mucosal lining, increasing hormone availability and reducing adrenal exhaustion. Doses of licorice root and gastrointestinal tract dietary supplements are typically between 500 milligrams and 1 gram.

Marshmallow Root

The root of the marshmallow plant has antihistamine and antioxidant properties. protects against stomach ulcers and promotes general digestive health.

Collagen Powder

Collagen and the amino acids proline and glycine found in bone broth are critical for healing a torn intestinal lining. Take 2 tablespoons of collagen protein twice daily, or drink 8–16 ounces of bone broth daily.

NAG

N-acetyl glucosamine's ability to preserve the stomach and intestines' lining has led to its recent popularity in conventional medicine. Osteoarthritis and inflammatory bowel diseases (IBDs), including ulcerative colitis and Crohn's disease, may benefit from NAG's anti-inflammatory properties.

Shilajit

The black, tar-like chemical has potent anti-inflammatory and gut-healing properties. With the help of shilajit, inflammation in the digestive tract can be minimized, and stomach ulcers can be prevented.

Reishi Mushrooms

Your gut houses a large portion of your immune system, which adaptogenic reishi mushrooms can help strengthen. Reishi not only aids in destroying disease-causing cells but also shields healthy genes from damage. In addition, Reishi helps your immune system because it aids the liver in its cleansing processes.

Lion's Mane Mushrooms

As a potent anti-inflammatory, lion's mane mushrooms may help your digestive system perform better. In a few scientific trials, the lion's mane mushroom has been demonstrated to prevent or reduce the size of stomach ulcers. Lab tests and preliminary research suggest that lion's mane may also dramatically relieve symptoms of gastritis and inflammatory bowel disease, two critical inflammatory disorders of the digestive tract.

FOODS TO AVOID FOR A HEALTHY GUT

Foods that are heavy in trans-saturated fat, low in beneficial nutrients, and capable of upsetting your gut bacteria balance are the worst choices. If you want a healthy digestive system, avoid these foods:

Red meat

Eating red meat regularly has been linked to increased N-nitroso compounds, gout flare-ups, gastrointestinal distress, and the overgrowth of gut bacteria. Heart disease and colon cancer are also more likely to develop. A dietitian might suggest switching to fish or plant-based proteins instead of red meat. Round, loin, and sirloin are healthier options than other cuts of beef.

Fried foods

By increasing the calorie density and degrading the oil, fried meals are unhealthy because they include more trans fats and fewer unsaturated fatty acids. In addition, fried meals can absorb heated oil, which has been shown to harm intestinal microbes. Thinking twice before buying fried foods is vital because they might cause an upset stomach.

Heavily processed foods

High levels of consumption of energy-dense and processed foods are characteristic of the Western diet and can be harmful to the gut microbiota. These items lack fiber and contain unhealthy ingredients like sugar and preservatives. A recent assessment found that eating a lot of ultra-processed food can change your gut bacteria and trigger inflammation.

Alcohol and other beverages

Regular alcohol consumption has been linked to alterations in the gut flora, which in turn have been associated with increased intestinal permeability and diarrhea. Caffeine in coffee, drinks, and chocolate can all contribute to an overly caffeinated system and subsequent diarrhea.

Dairy

Yogurt and kefir benefit gut microbes, but regular milk and cheese might be toxic. Full-fat coconut and almond milk are two options for lactose intolerant or allergic to dairy but still need a refreshing drink.

Fructose

Sucralose, saccharin, and polyols are only some of the artificial sweeteners that have been linked to altered bacterial colony populations and microbial makeup in the gut. Fructose, a fruit sugar, can disrupt the balance of good bacteria in the digestive tract. A microbial metabolite problem and gut dysbiosis were shown to result from the gut microbiome's conversion of fructose that was not absorbed into short-chain fatty acids (SCFAs), hydrogen, methane, and carbon dioxide.

EFFECTS OF ALCOHOL ON THE DIGESTIVE SYSTEM

In addition to raising one's risk of cancer and liver disease, heavy alcohol consumption can also harm one's digestive tract. The stomach, esophagus, liver, pancreas, intestines, mouth, throat, and anus are all components of your digestive system. Each organ has a specific role in taking in food, breaking it down, absorbing its nutrients, and flushing out waste.

The effects of alcohol on your digestive tract are as follows:

- **Your mouth and throat**: Saliva is a porous barrier, and alcohol quickly enters it, converting to acetaldehyde, which is toxic to oral tissues. One-third of all cases of mouth and throat cancer were linked to alcohol consumption. Furthermore, alcohol consumption may boost the risk of mouth cancer with smoking.

- **Your esophagus:** The long tube connecting your mouth and stomach is called the esophagus, and drinking alcohol can harm its cells and raise your risk of developing esophageal cancer once it has been swallowed. Cancer risk is increasing, and acid reflux contributes to that by damaging cells.

- **Your stomach:** Alcohol use has been linked to decreased acid production, mucous cell damage, and a prolonged emptying time in the stomach. A delay in stomach emptying due to inflammation and lesions might result in bacterial food spoilage and abdominal pain. Alcohol, whether consumed infrequently or frequently, can also disrupt digestive processes.

- **Your liver:** This vital organ's primary function is to flush harmful substances from the body. However, the liver processes alcohol in multiple ways, all of which produce acetaldehyde, a cell-damaging and inflammation-inducing byproduct of alcohol metabolism. The result can be increased liver fat production, a condition known as fatty liver disease. Toxic byproducts created during alcohol metabolism can also cause cell and tissue damage.

- **Your intestines**: Through the anus, alcohol reaches the big intestine, which may promote cancerous growth. Both light and heavy drinkers have an increased risk of colorectal cancer by 21 percent and 52 percent, respectively.

ANTIBIOTICS AND THE MICROBIOME: A DOUBLE-EDGED SWORD

Antibiotics usually function by eliminating bacteria or stopping their growth. Most antibiotics do not know the difference between beneficial and harmful germs. This implies that they threaten the beneficial bacteria in your digestive system. Antibiotics alter the intestinal flora of many people in a way that cannot be reversed.

Restoring Balance in Your Gut

Antibiotics should not be used unless necessary. If you've taken antibiotics recently and are dealing with the after-effects of an imbalanced digestive system, try the following:

Make sure you're eating a variety of whole, fiber-rich foods.

The most critical information is that reestablishing a healthy gut microbiota balance can be accomplished quickly and effectively by eating a diet rich in varied fiber from whole plant sources. People who consume a wide variety of plant foods every week have gut microbiomes that are more robust, diversified, and numerous. Strict elimination diets starve different microbiome residents, while high-fiber diets foster a diversified microbiome. Eat more of these:

- Beans, chickpeas, and lentils
- Avocados and other tropical fruits, in addition to berries, apples, melons, and citrus
- Vegetables, including in-season vegetables (squash, asparagus), root vegetables (broccoli, cauliflower), and root vegetables (beets, garlic, onions, sweet potatoes, and more).
- Oatmeal, whole wheat, and barley
- Cashews, almonds, peanuts, and walnuts
- Seeds, from whole pumpkin and sunflower to ground flax and chia.

Prebiotics help the good bacteria in your gut thrive.

Eating foods high in prebiotics can help strengthen beneficial, anti-inflammatory bacteria in the gut. Onions, barley, artichokes, garlic, whole wheat, jicama, and beans are just a few foods that naturally contain prebiotic fiber. Although inulin is prebiotic, many avoid it because of its gas-inducing properties. B-GOS or HMOs would be more acceptable.

Eat fewer processed foods to protect your gut microbiota and intestinal barrier.

Certain additives included in highly processed foods have raised concerns among researchers because of their potential to disrupt the delicate balance between the immune-cell-rich gut wall and the bacterial inhabitants of our microbiome. Synthetic flavors, colors, and stabilizers are among these additives.

Rebalance your lifestyle

The stomach affects Every area of health, just as the gut influences every aspect of health. For example, lifestyle choices, such as getting enough sleep and exercising frequently, can affect the health of the gut microbiota. The other puzzle components include getting enough sleep, dealing with stress, and working out regularly.

Let's have a peek at what the next chapter covers diets to stabilize your gut.

- Intermittent fasting
- The Ketogenic Diet
- Paleo Diet
- The Mediterranean Diet
- Elimination Diet

9

DIETS TO RESTORE YOUR GUT

Diets to Restore Your Gut: Going from 'Gut-Wrenching' to 'Gut-Restoring'—Bon Voyage to Tummy Troubles!

INTERMITTENT FASTING

The basic concept is to cycle through eating and fasting regularly. The 16/8 regimen is a common approach in which you consume all of your daily calories in a short time frame (say, from 10 a.m. to 6 p.m.) and then fast for the next 8 hours. The 5:2 method is another option: you cut back on calories for just two days a week while maintaining your typical healthy eating habits for the other five. Fasting (or calorie restriction) every other day is known as alternate-day fasting. Fasting of a specific type has been demonstrated to aid in weight loss.

The health of your digestive system can benefit from intermittent fasting.

The health benefits of intermittent fasting include weight loss and a reduced risk of metabolic and cardiovascular illnesses. Recent research suggests that by boosting taxonomic diversity and driving microbial remodeling, intermittent fasting can change the composition of the human gut microbiome. The family Lachnospiraceae, which is a member of the Clostridiales order and has advantageous metabolic and anti-aging properties, causes baryogenesis in the gut. The microbiota may be involved in fasting and calorie restriction's metabolic and health benefits.

Tips for Successful Intermittent Fasting for Women Over the Age of 50

Women over 50 can use these suggestions to establish a long-term IF routine.

Start slow

If you want to ease into intermittent fasting, skipping breakfast is an excellent place to begin. Start your fast by skipping both dinner and breakfast. A 12-hour overnight fast can be accomplished with just four hours of active fasting (not counting sleep). If you feel comfortable fasting overnight, you can move on to longer fasts.

Get enough calories

Most intermittent fasting studies let people eat as much as they want during the feeding periods. The vast majority of people will still reduce their caloric intake even under these lenient conditions. Extreme calorie restriction might have negative consequences. Maintaining a small caloric deficit of around 10% will help you avoid the negative consequences of calorie restriction, like exhaustion, sleep problems, and decreased muscle mass.

Prioritize protein

A diet that is low in protein exacerbates age-related muscle loss. Sarcopenia is a common problem among the elderly and a leading cause of disability. Consuming 100 grams of protein per day gets more difficult the longer you fast. For muscle preservation, a goal of 100 grams is reasonable.

Resistance train

Strength training is essential to complement IF. If you don't strength train, you lose muscle mass (lean mass) when fasting, and vice versa. As we get older, muscle is what keeps us moving. And as we age, upkeep becomes increasingly challenging. Avoid this by increasing your protein intake and weight lifting.

Get enough electrolytes

The loss of electrolytes like sodium and potassium increases while fasting. Electrolytes must be replenished to avoid headaches, weariness, and cramps. This includes adding salt to your food, eating foods high in electrolytes like spinach, and perhaps even taking an electrolyte supplement.

Consider a keto diet

Combining keto and IF can be an effective strategy for women over 50. Both plans can increase ketosis, decrease insulin, and kickstart weight loss. The keto diet has been studied and found to be effective for weight loss.

Eat a nutrient-dense diet

Since you'll be eating less frequently when using IF, making every meal matter is important. This calls for a diet rich in animal products, seafood, eggs, organ meats, produce, and heart-healthy fats. Instead of buying processed meals, focus on the outer aisles of the supermarket.

GUT MICROBIOME AND THE KETOGENIC DIET

The delicate ecosystem found in the gut significantly impacts your health. The brain and immune system, among others, rely on the assistance of these vital microbes to function properly. The bacteria in your stomach are also highly responsive to your food. Alterations to your regular diet can positively and negatively affect your microbiome's makeup and function.

The ketogenic diet is well known to cause significant changes to the gut microbiota by altering the metabolites that gut bacteria produce. Because of their potential impact on your health, it's important to understand how these alterations might improve or detract from the microbiome. Such factors can have an impact on the efficiency of several bodily systems, including the immune system, the brain, and the digestive system.

Positive Effects of the Ketogenic Diet on the Digestive Tract Microbiome

Boosts populations of good bacteria

Ketosis has been shown to augment the microbiome with bacteria involved in fat consumption and metabolism. These bacteria are helpful because they stimulate key immune cells and enhance the digestive processes already happening in the gut, both of which contribute to better overall health. Such organisms include Akkermansia, Firmicutes, Bacteroidetes, Lactobacillus, and Bacteroides.

Reduces the severity of several gastrointestinal and neurological diseases

The good bacteria in the gut microbiome that the ketogenic diet stimulates can help manage some neurological illnesses by increasing enzyme and hormone production. Conditions including epilepsy, seizures, autism, and Alzheimer's disease fall within this category. They help with insulin sensitivity, weight loss, and IBS symptoms.

Keto Diet

The ketogenic diet is a low-carb eating plan to keep the body in a metabolic state termed ketosis. The metabolic state of ketosis involves using fat for energy instead of glucose. On the ketogenic diet, ketosis is favored over refueling glycogen and protein stores. The staples of the ketogenic diet might surprise those who aren't accustomed to "high-fat" or "low-carb" diets.

Keto Food List

Here are some food items that are allowed and those that are not on the ketogenic diet:

Do not eat

- Cereals, bread, pasta, and other grain-based foods
- Honey, agave, maple syrup, and other sweeteners
- Fruit, like apples, bananas, oranges, and other varieties.
- Yams, potatoes, and other tubers

Do eat

- Meats, such as seafood, lamb, poultry, fowl, and eggs
- Vegetables that are low in carbohydrates, such as spinach, kale, and broccoli
- Hard cheeses, heavy cream, butter, and other forms of high-fat dairy products
- Macadamias, walnuts, sunflower seeds, and other nuts and seeds
- Avocados and berries (especially those with a minimal glycemic impact, such as blackberries and raspberries)
- Sugar substitutes, including stevia, erythritol, monk fruit, and others that are low in carbohydrates

- Saturated fats, trans fats, trans fatty acids, trans fatty acids, trans fatty acids, etc.

The Ketogenic Diet: An Overview

Reduce carbs while increasing vegetable intake

To enter ketosis, a very low-carb diet is required. For two weeks, a person must keep their net carb intake between 20 and 40 grams per day in order to enter ketosis. Consuming a diet high in ketogenic-supportive vegetables—such as kale, broccoli, spinach, asparagus, mushrooms, and peppers—is essential for entering the metabolic state of ketosis. Eating a diet high in whole foods and slowly introducing net carbs will help you avoid setbacks, hunger, and the need for processed foods. Recipes using low-carb alternatives are just as satisfying.

Decrease stress

If your job or personal life is more stressful than usual, you should wait to start a keto diet. The stress hormone cortisol, when present in excess, can cause an increase in blood sugar that impedes the body's transition toward ketosis. Getting enough shut-eye, working out frequently, and practicing stress-busting activities like yoga and meditation can all help. As an added bonus, make it a habit to get between seven and nine hours of sleep every night by maintaining a regular bedtime routine.

Increase healthy fats

Following a low-carb ketogenic diet, you eat more fat to compensate for the energy you're not getting from carbohydrates. Most people who try the ketogenic diet fall short of their fat intake goals because they have been told for so long to shun fat. Olive oil, avocado oil, coconut oil, cheese, eggs, almonds, and fish are excellent examples of the kinds of plant and animal fats that should make up the bulk of your diet.

Increase exercise

Increasing physical activity can aid weight loss efforts in the same way that a diet can. Regular exercise on the ketogenic diet helps hasten the process of entering ketosis and adapting to a low-carb, high-fat lifestyle. Because getting into ketosis requires ridding the body of all glucose, the more frequently you exercise, the sooner your body burns up its glycogen stores and switches to using fat for fuel. When first starting the ketogenic diet, you may experience fatigue. To help your body adjust to its new diet, start any new exercise routine slowly and do lots of low-intensity activities.

Increase your water intake

Because of their diuretic effects, low-carb diets like keto can deplete your body with the water necessary to sustain your metabolism and regular physiological functions. Constipation, dizziness, and cravings might result from not drinking enough water, especially during the induction phase. Make sure you're receiving enough electrolytes by eating some broth or salting your food a little more than usual, in addition to drinking plenty of water. You should also aim for six to eight glasses of water every day. If you've increased your workout intensity or it's a hot day, you should drink even more.

Maintain your protein intake

You need to consume enough protein on a ketogenic diet to supply your liver with the amino acids it needs to make new glucose for your kidneys and red blood cells, which cannot function on ketones or fatty acids. Not receiving enough protein can lead to muscle loss, while getting too much can prevent ketosis.

Keep up the electrolytes

Sodium, potassium, and magnesium are the three most abundant electrolytes in the human body. It's important to take in enough of these to prevent the temporary but annoying side effects.

Eat only when you are hungry

Don't feel obligated to eat a certain number of times each day or to nibble continually. Eating on a keto or low-carb diet too frequently is unnecessary and may prevent or slow down weight loss. Eat only if you're hungry; skip meals if you're not. Cutting back on carbs can help with this because doing so reduces hunger.

Maintain your social life!

When you first begin the ketogenic diet, you don't have to cook all of your meals at home. Check the menu in advance, inquire about the restaurant's nutritional information, order mostly meat, and vegetables, and choose a salad as a side dish instead of a starchy one, such as French fries.

THE MEDITERRANEAN DIET MAY HELP MAINTAIN A HEALTHY DIGESTIVE SYSTEM

Altering your food will always have an effect on the trillions of bacteria that call your gut home. The Mediterranean diet is rich in vitamins, phytochemicals, and fiber since it emphasizes the consumption of fresh, plant-based foods. These help beneficial germs like bacteria thrive in the gut, which is crucial to the micro-biome's operation. Many of these nutrients are also powerful antioxidants, warding off the harmful effects of stress on the microbiome in the body and the intestinal environment.

Improvements in Gut Microbiota with a Mediterranean Diet

Activates the saccharolytic metabolic pathway

The gut microbiota aids in the breakdown of macronutrients through the proteolytic and saccharolytic catabolic pathways. Both the proteolytic pathway, which results in metabolic products that can cause inflammation and leaky gut, and the saccharolytic pathway, which employs fermentation to break down sugars in carbs to provide energy, are important. For a more efficient and healthful breakdown of macronutrients, the Mediterranean diet promotes the saccharolytic pathway and the prevalence of saccharolytic microbial species in the gut.

Increased metabolic activity and diversity of beneficial bacteria

The Mediterranean diet is beneficial to the gut and microbiota in many ways due to the high concentration of plant-based vitamins and phytochemicals in this diet. This includes a rise in the number of healthy bacteria in the gut, such as bifidobacteria. In order to maintain a healthy immune system and a healthy digestive tract, bifidobacteria are crucial. The microbes in your gut produce and release important metabolites and vitamins thanks to this diet. Colon cells rely on metabolites such as short- and long-chain fatty acids for energy, and these metabolites play a vital role in maintaining the integrity of the intestinal barrier and regulating immune cell responses.

Reduction in intestinal inflammation

The Mediterranean diet is effective in reducing intestinal inflammation because it emphasizes particular foods and healthy lifestyle habits, such as regular physical activity. C-reactive protein and other inflammatory indicators have been shown to decrease within 6 weeks of following a Mediterranean-style diet. Inflammation is down in those who follow the Mediterranean diet, and with that comes a decrease in the prevalence of chronic diseases linked to inflammation and compromised microbiota. Diseases like Crohn's, UC (Ulcerative colitis), and IBS all fall into this category.

The Mediterranean Diet

Fruits, vegetables, whole grains, nuts, fish, seafood, olive oil, and red wine are the cornerstones of the Mediterranean diet. It includes moderate amounts of cheese, yogurt, red meat, and red wine while excluding processed foods, excessive saturated fat, trans fat, and refined sugar. It's a method of eating that prioritizes fresh, natural foods to curb cravings and keep you at a healthy weight and level of vitality. The tenets of the Mediterranean diet and way of life are as follows:

- Incorporate a wide range of fresh, whole foods into your diet
- Reduce your intake of sodium, refined sugar, saturated fat, and trans fat.
- Replace butter or margarine with olive oil.
- Maintain a daily exercise routine of at least 30 minutes.
- Abstain from smoking
- Limit portion size
- Drink an adequate amount of water
- Consume alcohol in moderation
- Relax, especially after meals
- Laugh, smile, and enjoy life.

Mediterranean Diet Pyramid

1. Non-refined whole grains like quinoa and brown rice are central to the Mediterranean diet, along with vegetables and fruits.
2. Olive oil is more beneficial than other vegetable oils and is a staple of the Mediterranean diet.

3. Protein-rich legumes, nuts, seeds, and lentils make a better and more satisfying meat alternative.

4. To add heat to a dish, mix herbs with olive oil and freshly cracked black pepper, or use curry powder.

5. Consuming fish and seafood regularly is crucial for one's mental and cardiovascular well-being.

6. A healthy diet must include poultry, eggs, cheese, and yogurt, but only in moderation.

7. Legumes, beans, and seeds can easily fill in the few servings of red meat that you should be eating each week.

8. The Mediterranean diet encourages moderate wine consumption—one glass per day.

9. Walking or bicycling to work are examples of the moderate physical activity and social connection that are hallmarks of the Mediterranean way of life. Family members take their time eating together, allowing for more conversation and enjoyment of the meal.

On the Mediterranean diet, you need to consume:

- At least 3 servings of fish and seafood per week
- Up to 4 servings of sweets per week
- 3 to 5 servings of whole grains per day

- 4 to 6 servings of healthy fats per day
- 3 to 5 servings of red meat per month
- Up to one 5-ounce glass per day
- 3 to 5 servings (2 eggs) per week
- At least 4 servings of fresh fruits and vegetables per day
- Up to 7 servings of dairy products per week
- 2 to 5 servings of poultry per week

PALEO DIET

The Paleo diet, known as the Paleolithic or Caveman diet, offers a compelling approach to support gut health for women over 50. Drawing inspiration from our ancestors' eating patterns, this dietary approach focuses on whole, unprocessed foods that align with our genetic makeup. Incorporating the principles of the Paleo diet into your lifestyle can nourish your gut, promote optimal digestion, and enhance overall well-being.

The Paleo diet's core lies in a foundation built on natural, nutrient-dense foods. Fresh fruits and vegetables, lean proteins, healthy fats, nuts, and seeds form the cornerstone of this way of eating. Embracing these natural, unprocessed foods provides your body with essential vitamins, minerals, and fiber, promoting gut health and a balanced microbiome.

One key aspect of the Paleo diet is the exclusion of grains and legumes. While these foods can be nutritious, they can also pose challenges for digestion, particularly for women over 50 who may experience age-related changes in their gastrointestinal system. You can alleviate digestive stress and support a healthier gut environment by eliminating grains and legumes containing potential gut irritants such as gluten and lectins.

Another advantage of the Paleo diet is its emphasis on eliminating refined sugars and processed foods. These dietary culprits can disrupt the delicate balance of the gut microbiome, contributing to inflammation, imbalances in gut bacteria, and digestive discomfort. By choosing whole, unprocessed foods, you reduce your intake of these gut-disrupting substances and provide a nourishing environment for your gut microbiome to thrive.

While the Paleo diet provides a solid framework for gut health, it's important to personalize it to your individual needs. As a woman over 50, you may have specific dietary requirements and considerations. Consulting with a healthcare professional or registered dietitian specializing in gut health can help you tailor the Paleo diet to suit your unique needs, ensuring you meet your nutritional requirements and achieve optimal gut wellness.

Remember, embracing the Paleo diet for gut health is not a one-size-fits-all approach. It is essential to listen to your body, make adjustments as needed, and be mindful of any food sensitivities or intolerances you may have. By adopting the principles of the Paleo diet and customizing it to your individual needs, you can tap into its potential to support gut health, improve digestion, and enhance your overall well-being as you navigate the transformative years of life over 50.

ELIMINATION DIET

As a diagnostic and therapeutic technique, an elimination diet can help identify foods contributing to IBS and other symptoms like skin rashes, joint discomfort, and mental fogginess.

What health issues might benefit from an elimination diet?

A wide range of health problems can benefit from an elimination diet. Let's take a look at the top three most-studied health issues:

IBS

Elimination diets have been beneficial for people with irritable bowel syndrome (IBS). Of all the elimination diets studied, the low-FODMAP diet has proven to be the most effective. Two systematic reviews found that following the diet improved quality of life by decreasing digestive symptoms and abdominal pain. Researchers have observed that people with irritable bowel syndrome (IBS) and inflammatory bowel disease (IBD) benefit from a low-FODMAP diet.

Autoimmune Diseases

Clinical trials of elimination diets for autoimmune illnesses have shown promising results. Experiments with c-reactive protein (the level of this protein rises with inflammation) reveal that an elimination diet reduces systemic inflammation.

Food Intolerances

An elimination diet is helpful for those with food intolerances, where the digestive system is unable to fully process certain foods. Some people have difficulty digesting carbohydrates known as lactose, histamine, fructose, and FODMAPs. Skin rashes, headaches, joint discomfort, and brain fog are just some of the symptoms that can result from not being able to digest certain foods or from the fermentation of certain foods (as is the case with fermentable oligosaccharides and monosaccharides, or FODMAPS).

How does it work?

There are two stages to an elimination diet: elimination and reintroduction.

The Elimination Phase

The elimination phase lasts for around two to three weeks, during which time you avoid eating foods you believe are worsening your illness. Do not eat anything if there is any doubt that doing so could make you ill. Some people have allergic reactions to foods like peanuts, tree nuts, corn, soy, dairy, wheat, gluten, citrus, pork, eggs, nightshade vegetables, and shellfish. Now is the time to investigate whether or not your diet may be to blame for your symptoms. After two to three weeks of avoiding the offending foods, you should see a doctor if your symptoms have not subsided.

The Reintroduction Phase

The second stage, known as reintroduction, involves gradually reintroducing previously avoided items back into the diet. While monitoring for reactions, gradually introduce each food category over the course of two to three days. Here are some signs to keep an eye out for:

- Difficulty sleeping
- Rashes and skin changes
- Stomach pain or cramps
- Changes in bowel habits
- Changes in breathing
- Bloating
- Joint pain
- Headaches or migraines
- Fatigue

If you reintroduce a food group and don't have any adverse reactions, you can safely continue eating that food group. However, if you see symptoms like the ones listed above, you have discovered a trigger item and should eliminate it from your diet. It usually takes about 5–6 weeks for the whole process to finish. Consult your physician or a registered nutritionist before making drastic dietary changes. A nutritional shortage may result from cutting out too many dietary types.

On an elimination diet, what foods are off-limits?

The most severe elimination diets have the highest success rates. During the elimination phase, the more foods you avoid, the more likely you are to figure out which ones are causing your symptoms. During the elimination phase, it is normal to avoid eating foods like:

- Don't eat any citrus fruits like oranges or grapefruits.
- White potatoes, tomatoes, cayenne pepper, peppers, eggplant, and paprika all belong to the family of vegetables known as nightshades, which you should avoid.
- Remove all nut and seed products from your diet.
- Remove all beans, lentils, peas, and soy-based items from your diet.
- Stay away from bread, pasta, cereal, and other starchy meals. It's best to stay away from gluten in any form.
- You should stay away from cold cuts, processed meats, cattle, poultry, pigs, eggs, and seafood, as well as fatty fish.
- Avoid milk, cheese, yogurt, and ice cream, along with all other dairy products.
- Butter, margarine, hydrogenated oils, mayonnaise, and spreads are examples of fats to stay away from.
- Stay away from alcoholic beverages, coffee, black tea, soda, and other caffeinated drinks.
- Avoid sauces, relish, and mustard if you can.

- Stay away from white and brown sugar, honey, and other sweeteners.
- Chocolate, sweets, maple syrup, corn syrup, agave nectar, high-fructose corn syrup, and a few other things

Other foods not on this list may also be problematic, so it's best to avoid them if you can.

The Elimination Diet: What Can You Eat?

An elimination diet may be restrictive, but it's still possible to eat well and enjoy it. These are examples of acceptable foods:

- Fruits: Almost all fruit, but avoid citrus fruits especially.
- Vegetables, with the exception of nightshades, include most vegetables.
- Grains such as rice and buckwheat.
- Wild game, turkey, lamb, and cold-water fish like salmon
- Coconut milk and unsweetened rice milk are two examples of dairy-free alternatives.
- Fats like coconut oil, flaxseed oil, and extra-virgin olive oil that have been cold-pressed
- Water and herbal teas.

- Fresh herbs, black pepper, spices (save for cayenne pepper and paprika), and apple cider vinegar are all examples of spices, condiments, and other items.

Create new recipes and experiment with herbs and spices to add taste without breaking your calorie restriction.

10

HARMONIZE YOUR DIGESTIVE HEALTH: ENHANCING GUT WELLNESS THROUGH YOGA

Yoga and the Gut: Where Downward Dog Meets Digestive Dialogue... Mind Over Munchies!

Many lifestyle disorders may be traced back to gut dysfunction, highlighting the importance of keeping your gut in good working condition. Yoga, a well-liked physical practice, benefits the digestive system. Vagal-nerve-stimulating asanas suit the digestive system, mood, and energy level. One's digestive and overall health can both benefit from regular yoga practice. Yoga poses like this are good for your digestive system.

BOAT POSE

The abdominal muscles are strengthened in the boat posture, which in turn improves digestion. As a bonus, it stimulates the production of enzymes that aid digestion. When held to its fullest potential, this pose helps to release tension in the abdomen and the liver.

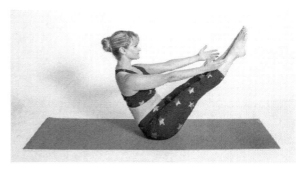

Photo Credit: www.yogajournal.com

How to do this pose:

1. Get down on all fours with your knees bent, feet flat on the floor, hands on your hips, and fingers pointing toward the floor.
2. To lengthen your spine, inhale and press your palms firmly into the ground.
3. Keep your hips planted on the ground and your spine in a neutral position as you slowly lift your torso back.

4. While keeping your knees bent, lift your feet off the floor until your shins are parallel to the floor.

5. Raise your arms so that they are perpendicular to the ground.

6. For a few seconds, hold this position.

7. Stand with your legs completely straight, creating a "V" shape with your body. Stay here for 2–5 deep breaths.

8. Exhale, then embrace your knees in a bear hug.

9. Take a deep breath, then drop your forehead to your knees while you straighten your spine.

10. Relax and take some deep breaths. Inhale deeply, raise your chin and exhale as you cross your legs.

11. Perform the full workout three to five more times.

SEATED FORWARD BEND POSES

The forward bend in a seated position aids digestion by stimulating the liver and kidneys. When we lean forward, our stomachs and pelvic organs take the brunt of the strain. The stimulation of your internal organs by this external stress promotes holistic healing. Try adopting this posture right before bedtime if you have difficulty relaxing and falling asleep.

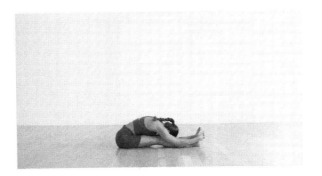

How to do the pose:

1. Root your tailbone to the floor as you sit.
2. Engage your leg muscles without making them overly stiff or rigid by stretching your legs straight in front of you.
3. Maintain knee strength and flexibility.
4. Raise your side arms over your head as you inhale deeply through your nostrils and exhale slowly through your mouth.
5. Reese your hips into the ground and slowly stoop so that your chest is between your knees. Avoid straining yourself too much on the first try. Instead, let your muscles warm up and loosen up throughout a series of reps.
6. Stretch your arms out straight and rest your hands on your legs, feet, or the floor while maintaining this squatting stance.

7. Stay here for as long as you feel safe doing so, breathing deeply and slowly.
8. Return to the starting position gradually and repeat the exercise several times.

CAMEL POSE

Camel's stance requires a lot of concentration. As soon as you release the stance, you'll start to experience the positive effects. Your digestive system will benefit from the camel stance since it improves your overall circulation. The elongation of the torso has a reawakening effect on the digestive system. The discomfort of heartburn is reduced as a side effect.

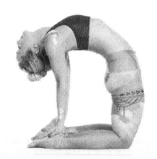

How to do the pose:

1. Bring your knees up to your shins on your yoga mat and place your hands there. Relax with a

pillow under your knees. The correct posture calls for a slight upward tilt of the shoulders and feet while keeping the knees straight.

2. Arc your back by drawing your tailbone toward your pubic bone, and bring your palms over your feet as you inhale. If you have problems getting up due to your hands, try curling your toes.

3. Put your head and shoulders back.

4. Hold this position and breathe normally for a bit. You can go back to square one as your exhalation continues.

WIND-RELIEVING POSE

As its name implies, the "wind-relieving pose" helps alleviate symptoms of bloating and flatulence. If you're having trouble passing gas, try striking this stance to calm your body, bowels, and intestines.

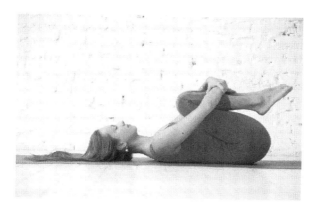

How to do the pose:

1. Both of your feet should lie flat on the ground, and your hands should be at your sides. Take a few deep breaths to calm down, and as you let out the last one, bring your right knee up to your chest.

2. While keeping your left leg straight, bring your right thigh toward your core using your hands on your shinbone. Relax your shoulders, sit up straight with your spine in a neutral position, and reach across your body to touch your right knee as you take a big breath in.

3. Don't rush. Just take a long breath or two and relax. As you let your breath out, slowly lower your body until you are back where you started. After completing the motion with your right and left legs, switch.

4. Calm yourself, take a few deep breaths, and do three or four sets.

SITTING HALF SPINAL TWIST

The half-spinal twist efficiently induces detoxification of the intestines by releasing toxins there in a tourniquet-like fashion. By stimulating blood flow to the abdominal region, twists have the effect of massaging the organs there. They are great for relieving constipation, bloating, and gas.

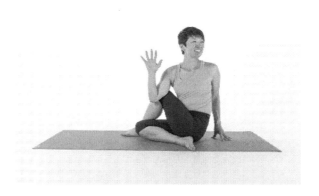

How to do the pose:

1. Sit up straight, propping your forearms on the floor or mat behind you.
2. Put your legs straight out in front of you and raise them.

3. Bend your right knee and step your right foot outside of your left knee to achieve this.

4. Breathe in deeply and lengthen your chest. As you exhale, rotate to the right and wrap your left arm over your right knee, or place the top part of your left arm on the outside of your right leg near the knee.

5. Maintain this position for a few breaths, expanding your upper back as you lift your chest with each inhalation and twisting your upper body slightly further with each exhalation.

6. Spin around till your front is facing you; then, spin around to your other side and repeat.

TRIANGLE POSE

The benefits of the triangle pose on digestion, appetite, and constipation are well documented. The kidneys and other abdominal organs are encouraged to function more efficiently by a combination of massage and increased blood flow to the area.

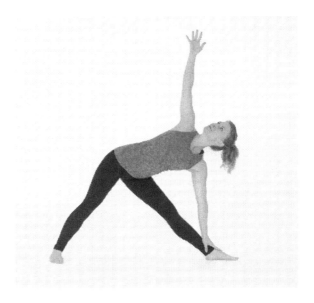

How to do the pose:

1. Standing with your feet slightly wider apart than your hips will give you the mountain stance. Your hands should be at about shoulder height.
2. Don't stop pushing forward as if nothing were wrong. Step 45 degrees to the left and bring your left heel toward your torso.
3. Balance yourself by putting the same amount of weight on each foot.
4. While taking deep breaths, bring your arms up to your shoulders and then down to your sides.

Take a big breath in a while, stretching your
right arm as far as it will go past your right foot.

5. Stretch out your left arm forward and into a
    plie position while placing your right hand on
    your right leg.

6. Face the extended arm and twist your upper
    body to face the short end of the mat. Avoid
    craning your neck by looking straight ahead.

7. Maintain for at least five full breaths, preferably
    more. Repeat on the other side.

CAT AND COW POSE

The cat and cow stance helps move food through the
digestive tract and relieves gas, bloating, and stress in
the stomach by opening the abdomen. Moreover, the
back discomfort and muscle strain that can occur from
not stretching your spine in both directions are
alleviated.

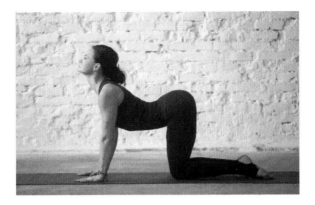

How to do the pose:

1. On your hands and knees, get on the floor in a countertop position.
2. Put your arms on the floor before your shoulders, look up slowly while taking a deep breath, and gently stretch your back. This stance is often called the "cat pose."
3. Round your back as you exhale, pulling your belly button against your spine, and glance down at your midsection.
4. The ruminant stance describes how you're lying here. Five to ten repetitions of cat and cow stances should be performed.

CHILD'S POSE

The child's posture is the most restorative because of the relaxing effect it has on the practitioner. This posture aids digestion by compressing the organs responsible for digestion. This pose can alleviate the symptoms of IBS and stomach ulcers by reducing stress.

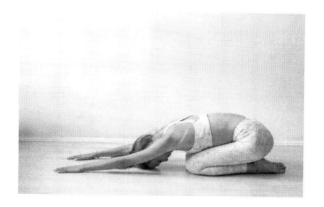

How to do the pose:

1. Put your hands on your knees and lean back on your heels without slouching forward. Relax your shoulders and stoop till your head touches the ground. Keep your knees bent and your ankles together.

2. Put your palms on the floor and your arms by your sides. Squeeze the upper body into the lower body gently.

3. Hold this position for five minutes while taking deep breaths. Raise your upper body, propped up by your forearms, as you take a deep breath.

4. Avoid straining your back by slowly rising from a lying position and sitting back down.

UPWARD-FACING DOG

Inversions like the upward dog are great for relieving abdominal pressure. The digestive organs are stimulated when the abdomen is opened. This is a helpful elimination posture since it relaxes the bowels and stimulates the intestines.

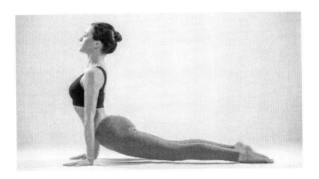

How to do the pose:

1. Lay down so that your tummy is flat.
2. Bend your elbows and bring your forearms close to your body. The shoulder blades tighten.
3. In an effort to pull your lower back up out of your pelvis, press the insides of your palms down slightly to the rear.
4. Maintain an upright, stiff stance with your legs and upper body off the ground. Lift your pelvis and glutes off the ground as you inhale and slowly raise your upper body. When leaning back, your neck shouldn't be strained.
5. Keep your arms and legs as straight as possible, and push off the balls of your feet to maximize your speed.
6. One to three deep breaths should be taken while holding this position. Relax your abs and slowly lie down on your back as you exhale.

CONCLUSION

EMBRACING THE JOURNEY TO GUT WELLNESS FOR WOMEN OVER 50

Embracing a Thriving Gut and Radiant Health: The Final Chapter. Spoiler Alert: It's a Gut-Busting Comedy of Digestive Triumphs!

The term "gut health" encompasses the intricate workings of our digestive tract, a complex system consisting of various organs responsible for breaking down food, absorbing nutrients, and eliminating waste. Beyond these functions lies the remarkable world of the gut microbiome, a diverse community of microorganisms that profoundly impacts our overall well-being. Achieving and maintaining a balanced gut microbiome is especially crucial for women over 50, as age-related changes in the gastrointestinal system can give rise to digestive issues and potential health complications.

The aging process brings shifts in the gut ecosystem, leading to discomforts, such as constipation, diarrhea, and an increased vulnerability to gastrointestinal problems. Recognizing the significance of gut health, women over 50 can take charge of their well-being by gaining knowledge about the factors influencing gut health and implementing strategies to enhance it.

Digestive issues extend beyond mere inconveniences; they can potentially undermine our overall health and happiness. Research has linked gastrointestinal disturbances to various health problems, including obesity, mood disorders, autoimmune conditions, and certain cancers. However, it is essential to remember that our gut health is not predetermined; we can improve it through education, awareness, and targeted interventions.

This comprehensive guide empowers women over 50 to reclaim control over their digestive system and embark on a transformative journey towards improved gut health. By understanding the origins of digestive problems, making informed dietary and lifestyle changes, and exploring natural therapies, readers will gain valuable insights and practical advice tailored specifically to their needs.

No longer should digestive woes hold you back from living your best life. This guide provides a roadmap to repair and optimize your digestive system, unlocking the potential for increased energy, radiant skin, and a renewed zest for life. It delves into the interconnectedness between gut health, hormone function, and weight regulation, offering valuable knowledge and inspiration for positive transformations.

With the wisdom and resources shared in this book, women over 50 can break free from the limitations of poor gut health. Discover the joy of guilt-free eating, boost your energy levels, and cultivate a positive body image. This guide equips you with the tools to navigate the intricacies of gut health, empowering you to embrace a longer, healthier, and more vibrant life.

So, let us embark on this transformative journey together, where knowledge becomes the catalyst for change and where a thriving gut paves the way to optimal well-being. Say goodbye to digestive distress and embrace a future filled with vitality, joy, and the freedom to savor life's every moment. The path to gut wellness awaits you.

REFERENCES

Henderson, R. (2018, May 31). *The digestive system.* https://patient.info/news-and-features/the-digestive-system

Your Digestive System & How it Works. (2023). *National Institute of Diabetes and Digestive and Kidney Diseases.* https://www.niddk.nih.gov/health-information/digestive-diseases/digestive-system-how-it-works

How Your Gut Health Affects Your Whole Body. (n.d.). WebMD. https://www.webmd.com/digestive-disorders/ss/slideshow-how-gut-health-affects-whole-body

The central role of the gut | Danone Research & Innovation. (n.d.). Danone Research & Innovation. https://www.danoneresearch.com/gut-and-microbiology/the-central-role-of-the-gut/

Becker, S., & Manson, J. E. (2020). Menopause, the gut microbiome, and weight gain: correlation or causation? *Menopause, 28*(3), 327–331. https://doi.org/10.1097/gme.0000000000001702

Gluck, S. (2020, June 29). *Hormones & Gut Health: The Estrobolome & Hormone Balance.* Marion Gluck. https://www.mariongluckclinic.com/blog/hormones-and-gut-health-the-estrobolome-and-hormone-balance.html

Restricted Content | The Institute for Functional Medicine. (2019, October 21). The Institute for Functional Medicine. https://www.ifm.org/restricted-content/

The Gut: Where Bacteria and Immune System Meet. (n.d.). https://www.hopkinsmedicine.org/research/advancements-in-research/fundamentals/in-depth/the-gut-where-bacteria-and-immune-system-meet

Chai, C. (2022, June 2). *Can a Healthier Gut Microbiome Boost Mood?* EverydayHealth.com. https://www.everydayhealth.com/emotional-health/can-a-healthier-gut-boost-your-mood/

Huang, T., Lai, J., Du, Y., Xu, Y., Ruan, L., & Hu, S. (2019). Current

Understanding of Gut Microbiota in Mood Disorders: An Update of Human Studies. *Frontiers in Genetics, 10.* https://doi.org/10.3389/fgene.2019.00098

Gora, A. (2022). Is there a link between gut health and weight loss? *livescience.com.* https://www.livescience.com/gut-health-and-weight-loss

Edermaniger, L. (2020). 9 Hard Facts About Your Gut Bacteria And Weight Loss. *Atlas Biomed Blog | Take Control of Your Health With Nononsense News on Lifestyle, Gut Microbes and Genetics.* https://atlasbiomed.com/blog/link-between-gut-bacteria-and-weight-loss/

Hewlett, A., DO. (2021, May 10). How your gut affects your whole body. *Nebraska Medicine Omaha, NE.* https://www.nebraskamed.com/gastrointestinal-care/how-your-gut-affects-your-whole-body

The importance of gut health | Parkview Health. (n.d.). Parkview. https://www.parkview.com/blog/the-importance-of-gut-health

Walker, S. (2021). 6 surprising health benefits of a healthy gut microbiome. *Healthista.* https://www.healthista.com/6-surprising-health-benefits-of-a-healthy-gut-microbiome/

Robertson, R., PhD. (2023, April 3). *How Does Your Gut Microbiome Impact Your Overall Health?* Healthline. https://www.healthline.com/nutrition/gut-microbiome-and-health

Robertson, R., PhD. (2020, August 20). *The Gut-Brain Connection: How it Works and The Role of Nutrition.* Healthline. https://www.healthline.com/nutrition/gut-brain-connection#TOC_TITLE_HDR_2

The Brain-Gut Connection. (2021, November 1). Johns Hopkins Medicine. https://www.hopkinsmedicine.org/health/wellness-and-prevention/the-brain-gut-connection

Cassano, O. (2023). Gut-Brain Connection: What It Is, Mental Health, and Diet. *joinzoe.com.* https://joinzoe.com/learn/gut-brain-connection

Harvard Health. (2021, April 19). *The gut-brain connection.* https://www.health.harvard.edu/diseases-and-conditions/the-gut-brain-connection

The surprising link between your microbiome and mental health. (n.d.). https://www.optum.com/health-articles/article/healthy-mind/

surprising-link-between-your-microbiome-and-mental-health/

Resetting the Hype Around the Vagus Nerve. (n.d.). Office for Science and Society. https://www.mcgill.ca/oss/article/critical-thinking/reset ting-hype-around-vagus-nerve

Professional, C. C. M. (n.d.). *Vagus Nerve.* Cleveland Clinic. https://my. clevelandclinic.org/health/body/22279-vagus-nerve

Seladi-Schulman, J., PhD. (2023, February 14). *What is the Vagus Nerve?* Healthline. https://www.healthline.com/human-body-maps/vagus-nerve

Han, Y., Wang, B., Gao, H., He, C., Hua, R., Liang, C., Zhang, S., Wang, Y., Xin, S., & Xu, J. (2022). Vagus Nerve and Underlying Impact on the Gut Microbiota-Brain Axis in Behavior and Neurodegenerative Diseases. *Journal of Inflammation Research, Volume 15,* 6213–6230. https://doi.org/10.2147/jir.s384949

The Brain-Gut Connection. (2021b, November 1). Johns Hopkins Medicine. https://www.hopkinsmedicine.org/health/wellness-and-prevention/the-brain-gut-connection

Harvard Health. (2021b, April 19). *The gut-brain connection.* https://www.health.harvard.edu/diseases-and-conditions/the-gut-brain-connection

How You Can Repair Your Vagus Nerves – Caring Medical Florida. (n.d.). https://www.caringmedical.com/can-repair-vagus-nerves/

Schneider, K. (2023, April 28). 5 Ways To Stimulate Your Vagus Nerve. *Cleveland Clinic.* https://health.clevelandclinic.org/vagus-nerve-stimulation/

MacGill, M. (2023, February 15). *What are the gut microbiota and human microbiome?* https://www.medicalnewstoday.com/articles/307998

Valdes, A. M., Walter, J., Segal, E., & Spector, T. D. (2018). Role of the gut microbiota in nutrition and health. *BMJ,* k2179. https://doi.org/10.1136/bmj.k2179

Robertson, R., PhD. (2023b, April 3). *How Does Your Gut Microbiome Impact Your Overall Health?* Healthline. https://www.healthline.com/nutrition/gut-microbiome-and-health#TOC_TITLE_HDR_5

Ferranti, E. P., Dunbar, S. B., Dunlop, A. L., & Corwin, E. J. (2014). 20 Things You Didn't Know About the Human Gut Microbiome.

Journal of Cardiovascular Nursing, 29(6), 479–481. https://doi.org/ 10.1097/jcn.0000000000000166

Well+Good. (2022). If You're a Woman, Here's Why Your Gut Issues Aren't Just in Your Head. *Well+Good.* https://www.wellandgood. com/womens-gut-health-renew-life/

Department of Health & Human Services. (n.d.). *Healthcare decision-making – options, benefits and risks.* Better Health Channel. https:// www.betterhealth.vic.gov.au/health/servicesandsupport/health care-decision-making-options-benefits-and-risks

Bigley II, J. (2022, March 14). What Are Prebiotics and What Do They Do? *Cleveland Clinic.* https://health.clevelandclinic.org/what-are-prebiotics/

Collins, J. (2019, August 5). *Prebiotics.* WebMD. https://www.webmd. com/digestive-disorders/prebiotics-overview

Murdock, S. (2023). How Hydration Affects Your Gut Health. *Pendulum.* https://pendulumlife.com/blogs/news/how-hydration-affects-your-gut-health

Prados, A. (2022). Is water the forgotten nutrient for your gut micro-biota? *Gut Microbiota for Health.* https://www.gutmicrobiotaforhealth. com/is-water-the-forgotten-nutrient-for-your-gut-microbiota/

Worst Foods for Digestion. (n.d.). WebMD. https://www.webmd.com/ digestive-disorders/ss/slideshow-foods-to-avoid

Food Diary - How to Keep Track of What You Eat. (2023, May 10). www.-heart.org. https://www.heart.org/en/healthy-living/healthy-eating/eat-smart/nutrition-basics/food-diary-how-to-keep-track-of-what-you-eat

Professional, C. C. M. (n.d.-a). *Probiotics.* Cleveland Clinic. https://my. clevelandclinic.org/health/articles/14598-probiotics

The Editors of Encyclopaedia Britannica. (1998, July 20). *Lactobacillus | bacteria.* Encyclopedia Britannica. https://www.britannica.com/ science/Lactobacillus

Duggal, N. (2017, April 15). *Bifidobacterium Bifidum: Benefits, Side Effects, and More.* Healthline. https://www.healthline.com/health/bifidobac terium-bifidum

What Are Probiotics? (n.d.). WebMD. https://www.webmd.com/diges tive-disorders/what-are-probiotics

Clt, E. J. M. R. (2023, February 16). *5 Possible Side Effects of Probiotics.* Healthline. https://www.healthline.com/nutrition/probiotics-side-effects

Dooley, B. (2021). 4 Ways To Reduce Stress for a Happier Gut. *Gastroenterology Consultants of San Antonio.* https://www.gastro consa.com/4-ways-to-reduce-stress-for-a-happier-gut/

Breathing Exercises to Improve Your Digestive Health | Blog | Loyola Medi- cine. (n.d.). Loyola Medicine. https://www.loyolamedicine.org/ about-us/blog/how-breathing-exercises-relieve-stress-and-improve-digestive-health

Insight Network, Inc. (n.d.). *Insight Timer - #1 Free Meditation App for Sleep, Relax & More.* Insight Network, Inc. Copyright (C) 2021. https://insighttimer.com/marnstein/guided-meditations/mindful ness-and-relaxation-for-gut-health

Insight Network, Inc. (n.d.-b). *Insight Timer - #1 Free Meditation App for Sleep, Relax & More.* Insight Network, Inc. Copyright (C) 2021. https://insighttimer.com/celiaroberts/guided-meditations/medita tion-on-gut-brain-connection

Let Nature Support Your Microbiome. (2022, June 7). UMass Chan Medical School. https://www.umassmed.edu/nutrition/blog/blog-posts/2022/4/let-nature-support-your-microbiome/

4 ways your environment could impact your gut health | Microba. (n.d.). Microba. https://insight.microba.com/blog/4-ways-your-living-environment-could-be-impacting-your-gut-health/

Team, S. Y., & Team, S. Y. (2021). The Gut-Sleep Connection: How To Heal Your Gut For Better Sleep. *MySlumberYard.* https://myslumber yard.com/blog/the-gut-sleep-connection/

Humphreys, C. (2020). Intestinal Permeability. In *Elsevier eBooks* (pp. 166-177.e4). https://doi.org/10.1016/b978-0-323-43044-9.00019-4

Suni, E., & Suni, E. (2023). Sleep Hygiene. *Sleep Foundation.* https:// www.sleepfoundation.org/sleep-hygiene

Key, A. P. (2019, November 19). *What Are Digestive Enzymes?* WebMD. https://www.webmd.com/diet/what-are-digestive-enzymes

Digestive Enzymes and Digestive Enzyme Supplements. (2022, February 10). Johns Hopkins Medicine. https://www.hopkinsmedicine.org/health/wellness-and-prevention/digestive-enzymes-and-digestive-enzyme-supplements

Ms, H. P. (2023, February 23). *11 Probiotic Foods That Are Super Healthy.* Healthline. https://www.healthline.com/nutrition/11-super-healthy-probiotic-foods

17 Probiotic Foods for Better Gut Health and More - Dr. Axe. (2023, June 14). Dr. Axe. https://draxe.com/nutrition/probiotic-foods/

Rd, A. S. M. (2021, May 11). *The 19 Best Prebiotic Foods You Should Eat.* Healthline. https://www.healthline.com/nutrition/19-best-prebiotic-foods

Cadman, B. (2018, October 1). *What prebiotic foods should people eat?* https://www.medicalnewstoday.com/articles/323214

Massy, H. (2022). 16 Great Foods for Prebiotics. *joinzoe.com.* https://joinzoe.com/learn/prebiotic-foods

Ms, E. L. (2019, February 26). *Leaky Gut Supplements: What You Need to Know to Feel Better.* Healthline. https://www.healthline.com/health/digestive-health/leaky-gut-supplements

Probiotics, L. (2020). 13 Foods That Are Terrible For Your Gut Health. *LoveBug Probiotics USA.* https://lovebugprobiotics.com/blogs/news/13-foods-that-are-terrible-for-your-gut-health

Probiotics, L. (2020b). 13 Foods That Are Terrible For Your Gut Health. *LoveBug Probiotics USA.* https://lovebugprobiotics.com/blogs/news/13-foods-that-are-terrible-for-your-gut-health

Castaneda, R., & Howley, E. K. (2023, January 18). Worst Foods for Gut Health. *US News & World Report.* https://health.usnews.com/wellness/food/slideshows/worst-food-for-gut-health?slide=4

Long Term Effects Of Alcohol Abuse On Health | Alcohol Think Again. (n.d.). Alcohol Think Again. https://alcoholthinkagain.com.au/alcohol-and-your-health/long-term-health-effects/digestive-system

Gouveia, A., & Gouveia, A. (2021). 6 Ways Alcohol Can Damage Your

Gut | UNC Health Talk. *UNC Health Talk.* https://healthtalk. unchealthcare.org/6-ways-alcohol-can-damage-your-gut/

Krans, B. (2021, October 21). Antibiotics Can Kill Healthy Gut Bacteria: Here's What to Eat to Counter That. *Healthline.* https://www. healthline.com/health-news/antibiotics-can-kill-healthy-gut-bacteria-heres-what-to-eat-to-counter-that

Intermittent fasting and the gut microbiome | Microba. (n.d.). Microba. https://insight.microba.com/blog/what-science-says-about-intermittent-fasting-and-the-gut-microbiome/

mindbodygreen. (2022, June 22). *Exactly How To Use Intermittent Fasting To Lose Weight & Heal Your Gut.* Mindbodygreen. https://www.mindbodygreen.com/articles/how-to-heal-your-gut-with-intermittent-fasting

What to Know About Intermittent Fasting for Women After 50. (2021, March 22). WebMD. https://www.webmd.com/healthy-aging/what-to-know-about-intermittent-fasting-for-women-after-50

Stanton, B. (2022). Intermittent Fasting for Women Over 50: 7 Tips for Success. *Carb Manager.* https://www.carbmanager.com/article/ygj3x heaaawus2xa/intermittent-fasting-for-women-over-50-7-tips-for/

University of California San Francisco. (2020, May 18). Ketogenic Diets Alter Gut Microbiome in Humans, Mice | UC San Francisco. *Ketogenic Diets Alter Gut Microbiome in Humans, Mice | UC San Francisco.* https://www.ucsf.edu/news/2020/05/417466/ketogenic-diets-alter-gut-microbiome-humans-mice

Rd, R. a. M. (2019, July 12). *Does Keto Affect Your Gut Health?* Healthline. https://www.healthline.com/nutrition/keto-and-gut-health

Clarke, C. (2022, September 25). *How To Start A Keto Diet [The Exact Plan To Follow For Beginners].* Ruled Me. https://www.ruled.me/how-to-start-a-keto-diet/

Merra, G., Noce, A., Marrone, G., Cintoni, M., Tarsitano, M. a. A., Capacci, A., & De Lorenzo, A. (2020). Influence of Mediterranean Diet on Human Gut Microbiota. *Nutrients, 13*(1), 7. https://doi.org/10.3390/nu13010007

How Does the Mediterranean Diet Affect Your Gut Microbiome? (2022, June

23). BIOHM Health. https://www.biohmhealth.com/blogs/health/how-does-the-mediterranean-diet-affect-your-gut-microbiome

BSc, K. G. (2023, May 17). *Mediterranean Diet 101: A Meal Plan and Beginner's Guide.* Healthline. https://www.healthline.com/nutrition/mediterranean-diet-meal-plan

Rd, R. R. M. (2017, July 2). *How to Do an Elimination Diet and Why.* Healthline. https://www.healthline.com/nutrition/elimination-diet

Chai, C. (2022b, June 2). *Why Exercise Is Good for Gut Health.* Everyday-Health.com. https://www.everydayhealth.com/fitness/can-exercise-boost-my-gut-health/

Pratt, E. (2018, September 24). Research Says Exercise Also Improves Your Gut Bacteria. *Healthline.* https://www.healthline.com/health-news/exercise-improves-your-gut-bacteria

User, G. (2021). 5 Exercises that Aid in Optimal Digestive Health | GHA. *Gastroenterology HealthCare Associates.* https://www.giwebmd.com/blog/2021/5/25/5-exercises-that-aid-in-optimal-digestive-health

Chai, C. (2022c, June 2). *Why Exercise Is Good for Gut Health.* Everyday-Health.com. https://www.everydayhealth.com/fitness/can-exercise-boost-my-gut-health/

Vlce, K. a. M. C. (2023). 8 Everyday Ways to Improve Your Gut Health Naturally. *Real Simple.* https://www.realsimple.com/how-to-improve-gut-health-naturally-6833619

Vagus Nerve. (n.d.-c). Physiopedia. https://www.physio-pedia.com/Vagus_Nerve

Missimer, A. (2021). How Your Vagus Nerve Affects Your Gut Health. *The Movement Paradigm.* https://themovementparadigm.com/how-your-vagus-nerve-affects-your-gut-health/

Devcich, A. (2022, August 1). Does Vagus Nerve Influence Gut Health? 4 Simple Hacks to Improve. *Gut Health & Complementary Therapies Clinic, Auckland.* https://www.houseofhealth.co.nz/vagus-nerve-gut/

Missimer, A. (2021b). How Your Vagus Nerve Affects Your Gut Health. *The Movement Paradigm.* https://themovementparadigm.com/how-your-vagus-nerve-affects-your-gut-health/

17535366R00133